THIS BOOK BELONGS TO
The Library of

....

....

©COPYRIGHT 2024

The content contained within this book may not be reproduced, duplicated, or transmitted without direct written permission from the author or the publisher. Under no circumstances will any blame or legal responsibility be held against the publisher, or author, for any damages, reparation, or monetary loss due to the information contained within this book. Either directly or indirectly.

Legal Notice:
This book is copyright protected. This book is only for personal use. You cannot amend, distribute, sell, use, quote, or paraphrase any part, or the content within this book, without the consent of the author or publisher.

Disclaimer Notice:
Please note the information contained within this document is for educational and entertainment purposes only. All effort has been executed to present accurate, up-to-date, and reliable, complete information. No warranties of any kind are declared or implied. Readers acknowledge that the author is not engaging in the rendering of legal, financial, medical, or professional advice. The content within this book has been derived from various sources. Please consult a licensed professional before attempting any techniques outlined in this book. By reading this document, the reader agrees that under no circumstances is the author responsible for any losses, direct or indirect, which are incurred as a result of the use of the information contained within this document, including, but not limited to — errors, omissions, or inaccuracies.

Thank you for Purchasing my book and taking the time to read it from front to back. I am always grateful when a reader chooses my work and I hope you enjoyed it!

With the vast selection available online, I am touched that you chose to be purchasing my work and take valuable time out of your life to read it. My hope is that you feel you made the right decision.

I very much would like to know what you thought of the book. Please take the time to write an honest and informative review on Amazon.com. Your experience and opinions will be of great benefit to me and those readers looking to make an informed choice.

With much thanks.

Table of Contents

Chapter 1: What Is Alzheimer's Disease? — 8

Chapter 2: What Is Caregiving? — 33

Chapter 3: Building Your Support Team — 50

Chapter 4: Mastering Communication With Healthcare Professionals — 60

Chapter 5: Navigating Legal and Financial Hurdles — 76

Chapter 6: Finding Your Peace — 91

Chapter 7: Is There Hope? — 107

Chapter 8: Creating Experiences — 124

Conclusion — 141

Introduction

I stared across the room, numb and unspeaking, drifting away from all that surrounded me for an entire ten minutes. As hard as I tried not to, I felt the inevitable tears well up in my eyes. I wanted to feel, scream, or take a break, if only for a fleeting moment of freedom. Every fiber of my being is in utter and complete exhaustion. In each moment that passed, I experienced varying emotions, from crying to laughing back to crying. I was exhausted from trying to constantly stay one step ahead of the current situation but felt I was always losing the battle. Everything I had held close to my heart for my future; the large family gatherings over a home-cooked meal, the housewarming, bridal and baby showers, and so much more was gone. At least that's how I felt before I discovered what I know now.

All the research you have conducted, the books and advice combined, is not enough to repaint forgotten memories and ease the sense of hopelessness. As you travel down this road, there comes a point when your energy crumbles, and you cannot go any further. Your mind becomes overwhelmed, your body gets tired, and you despair. It becomes challenging to determine the exact cause of your exhaustion, but worse than that, regaining hope and getting back on your feet seems almost unattainable.

It is not a matter of speed or distance covered. This is about navigating your new normal and taking on new responsibilities, such as ensuring your Loved One (LO) has the support they need to manage their diagnosis. This includes everything from attending appointments on time, helping with their finances, and calming them down when they get anxious in unfamiliar places. How many versions of the same story can you repeat every time your LO drifts out of themself and returns with no recollection of your previous conversation? What about the plans you had for your future; how have they changed? Or should we talk about the constant fear that something could happen to your LO if you left them home alone to work or fulfill other out-of-home commitments?

I understand what you are going through, the inevitable struggle, unnecessary pain, and countless sacrifices. This Book equips you with the fundamental tools to actively take care of your LOs when they need you the most. This book gives you the strength to stand tall when faced with the demanding requirements and heart-shattering obstacles of caregiving. You require incredible and relentless compassion to survive your new caregiving realities while giving your LOs the attention they need.

In *This Book*, you will learn:

- Roles and responsibilities of a caregiver
- How to balance your personal life with caregiving commitments
- Practical steps to maintaining peace while avoiding burnout
- Tips for stress-free interaction with doctors, lawyers, authority figures, and financial professions
- Simple ideas for engaging activities you can do together to create long-lasting experiences

With a subject as broad and complex as this one, we must start from the beginning before diving into caregiving. You should understand what you are dealing with before you dedicate yourself to caring for a LO who suffers from Alzheimer's Disease through the stages. Toward that, this book also reveals:

- The relationship between Alzheimer's disease and dementia

- Fiction and facts that commonly arise with the discussion of dementia and Alzheimer's disease versus typical signs of aging
- Signs and symptoms that manifest during the early stages of Alzheimer's disease
- Helpful statistics on Alzheimer's disease

And much more.

I organized this book so that you can take from it what you need when you need it. From understanding what the diagnosis entails, the roles and responsibilities of caregiving, and a host of helpful strategies, This Book equips you with the tools to understand early-onset Alzheimer's disease and the strength to care for your LOs without overworking yourself.

If that sounds like something you need, this is the book you want to hold close so that you do not stumble and fall into a deep cavern of hopelessness.

Chapter 1:

What Is Alzheimer's Disease?

One of my biggest struggles is not remembering the simple things: a name, a single word, or even where I've put my keys. I get so frustrated because the answer is RIGHT THERE, and I just can't pull it. I just wish my brain would act right.

—Mom

Every day that passes, we eat, drink, work, play, breathe, and love, and we turn another page in the chapters of our lives. As those chapters come close to an inevitable end, we all go through changes that differ from person to person. That is the process of aging. Although some of us may approach it with resistance, the process is unavoidable, with no respect to gender, location, or race. Because of the aging process, we can look back at our childhood days and laugh at our decisions, the good, the bad, and the ugly.

Normal Aging

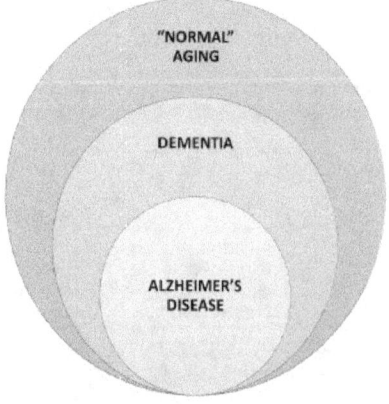

How do forgetfulness, gray hair, mood fluctuations, and changes in food preferences differ from signs of dementia? Significantly. There is a broad line between normal aging and dementia, and every caregiver should learn the difference to spot when these signs cross the line. Listed are some of the effects of "normal" aging:

- reduced functional capacity of organs
- slowed cell division
- reduced cardiac efficiency
- the gradual buildup of fat in arteries
- reduced hearing capacity
- weakened bones
- reduced joint flexibility
- slowed metabolism
- gradual death of nerve cells in the spinal cord and brain
- reduced eyesight
- constipation
- reduced skin elasticity
- urinary incontinence
- slowed nail growth
- loss of hair color and increased hair loss
- increased susceptibility to diseases and infections
- weight loss

What to do About it

Although we cannot stop or pause aging, making lifestyle changes helps reduce our risk for conditions and diseases that become common in old age. The following tips may help improve the quality of life for both you and your LO.

Exercise

When some people hear about exercise, they think about heavy workouts for weight loss, but the benefits of living an active life extend to mental fitness. Mental and physical activities improve heart and brain health, among other advantages.

Balance Your Diet

He who eats right extends his life expectancy. It's as simple as that. Vegetables, lean protein, fruits, healthy fats, and whole grains provide a lifelong subscription to healthy living. A nutrient-rich diet shields you from the wrath of various health hazards. Avoid processed foods as they may contain harmful substances. Find a way around trans fats and hydrogenated oils because the processes they go through to extend shelf life diminish their quality, making them unhealthy.

Socialize

Invite those old friends over and tease each other over childish mistakes from a long-buried past! When they leave, and you are alone again, those memories shape a priceless smile in place of a miserable countenance. People who choose to be alone often overthink their past, present, and future instead of *living*. When you build a social network; create new friendships while maintaining ties with friends and family, you reduce stress levels and slow aging.

Visit Your Doctor

At any life stage, strive to make medical consultations a habit. Visiting your doctor helps keep your overall health in check. As you grow older, you may want to control your blood pressure levels, improve bone health, and many other changes. The good news is: You can now visit your doctor without leaving the warmth of your home!

Dementia

As we age, we go through a series of changes. One of these changes is a loss of brain neurons, a change that also occurs in individuals with dementia. The speed at which healthy individuals lose neurons draws the line between normal aging and dementia.

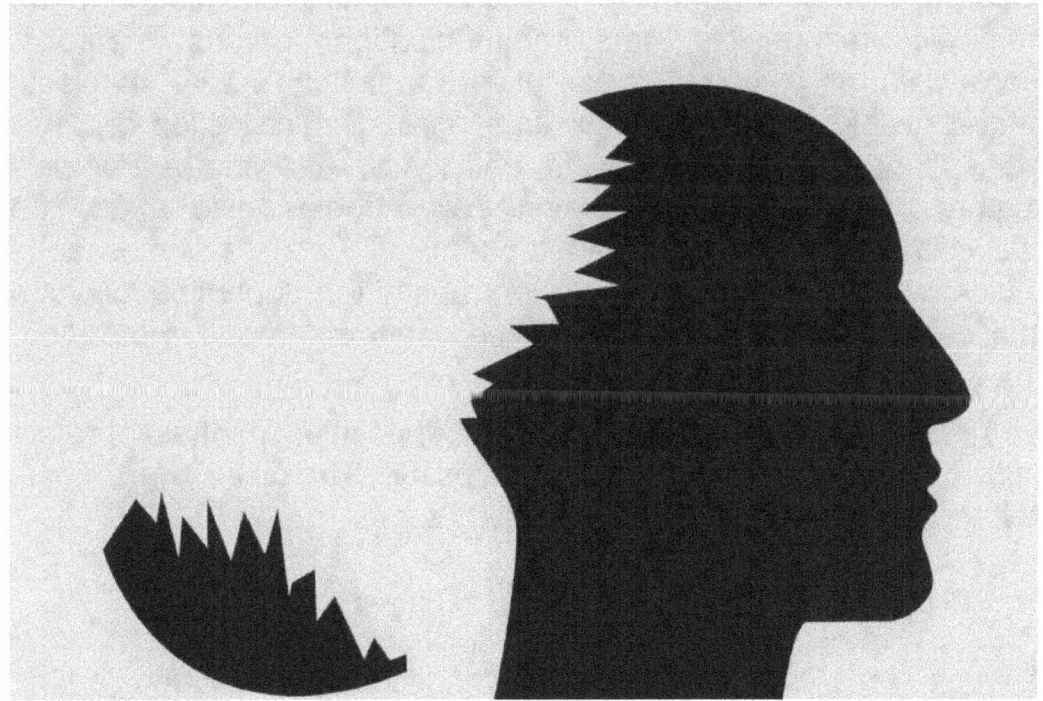

Dementia describes persistent conditions that interfere with normal mental processes, causing decreased cognitive function. It ranges from a point where it affects an individual's normal function, interfering with daily activities, to an extent when the afflicted individual can only depend on those around them for basic living needs.

Apart from aging, several other factors can cause dementia, including brain injuries. It is also important to know that not everyone with dementia has Alzheimer's disease. Before diving into Alzheimer's disease specifically, it is important to note several other forms of dementia.

Lewy Body Dementia

A buildup of protein bodies called Lewy bodies blocks the brain from producing sufficient amounts of certain neurotransmitters, brain chemicals responsible for communication among neurons. *Acetylcholine* is the chief chemical in transmitting nerve impulses, contraction of smooth muscles, and more. The collection of Lewy bodies causes an acetylcholine deficiency, affecting a person's memory and learning processes. Lewy bodies also affect the production of *dopamine*, another chemical that relays messages between brain neurons. The neurotransmitter dopamine plays a significant role in regulating one's sleep patterns, mood, motivation, etc.

Lewy body dementia stems from the deposition of these protein bodies, causing degeneration of brain tissue. The disease manifests itself through some of the following symptoms.

Sleep Difficulties

Although sleep challenges may go unnoticed by other people who are not close to the patient, these are common in individuals with

Lewy body dementia. Some obstacles are easy to manage, but others require specialized intervention from knowledgeable healthcare professionals.

- insomnia
- REM sleep disorder
- restless leg syndrome
- increased daytime sleepiness

Mood and Behavioral Fluctuations

Patients with Lewy Body disease may show negative changes in behavior and mood, and these changes worsen as the disease progresses. Some of these changes in behavior and mood include:

- extreme distrust of the surrounding people
- depression
- reduced interest in usual events or activities or events
- signs of paranoia such as suspecting that people are hiding things or talking behind their back
- less motivation for social interaction
- delusions, or firm opinions and beliefs that lack evidence
- restlessness or agitation and similar habits that include irritability, repeating words or phrases, and pacing
- anxiety and feeling disturbed in the absence of a LO

Movement Challenges

While some patients with Lewy body dementia may experience movement problems in the early stages of the disease, others may not have these until several years afterward. Signs of movement difficulties may start as minor changes in handwriting, then progress to apparent symptoms such as tremors and challenges in walking. Without proper diagnosis, minor signs of movement challenges in Lewy body dementia are easy to miss. Hence, it is crucial to know various other symptoms that signal disturbed movement in patients with Lewy body dementia.

- swallowing difficulties
- muscle stiffness or rigidity
- trouble balancing and repeatedly falling
- slow movement, frozen stance, or shuffling walk
- loss of coordination
- illegible handwriting
- shaking or tremors even in a relaxed state
- reduced facial expression
- stooped posture

Other Symptoms

Individuals suffering from Lewy body dementia can also experience significant changes in the part of the brain that regulates functions such as those of the muscles, heart, and glands. The patient may experience:

- fainting
- blood pressure problems
- body temperature fluctuations
- dizziness

In its early stages, this form of dementia can be challenging to diagnose, so doctors first carry out routine tests to rule out other health conditions that have similar symptoms. If, after routine tests, the healthcare providers have reason to suspect dementia, then they will perform further tests to evaluate the patient's cognitive functioning.

Several drugs help keep symptoms in check. Depending on the symptoms in question, one may require medicines to improve their movement, ease sleep, or drugs that work on thinking issues. Some lifestyle changes, such as eating healthy foods, practicing better sleeping habits, and exercising regularly, help patients cope better with the disease.

Frontotemporal Dementia

As the name suggests, Frontotemporal Dementia is another neurodegenerative disease caused by damage to the temporal and frontal lobes of the brain.

Located close to the temples, the temporal lobe plays a vital role in acquiring memory, processing sensory input, perception, etc. Significant damage to the temporal lobes can cause speech and spatial reasoning problems. The frontal lobe controls executive functions such as planning and decision making, as well as emotional regulation. It also manages operations related to communication, concentration, and consciousness. Each side of the temporal lobe handles the opposite side of the body; that is, damage on the right side of the temporal lobe would manifest on the left side of the body.

The signs and symptoms of this disease vary based on which side of the frontal or temporal lobe suffered damage. They usually progress at a steady rate, but sometimes, because of various factors, symptoms may worsen rapidly. Frontotemporal dementia presents itself in the forms listed next.

Behavioral Variant Frontotemporal Dementia

This form of frontotemporal dementia involves changes in behavior, judgment, and personality. Frontotemporal dementia patients may show difficulties with cognition, but their memory may remain unaffected.

Symptoms include:

- problems in organizing and prioritizing activities or tasks
- trouble with planning and sequencing events or steps
- saying or doing the same things repeatedly
- reduced interaction with family
- doing or saying inappropriate things without considering how the people around may interpret such behavior
- movement and language problems over time
- losing interest in activities they once enjoyed

Primary Progressive Aphasia (PPA)

Changes in communication skills are common in this form of frontotemporal dementia. Patients find it difficult to use language to write, read, speak, or understand general conversations. Challenges with judgment, memory, and reasoning may not manifest right initially, but they usually develop with time.

To better understand the symptoms of primary progression, we can categorize it into three classes as follows:

Semantic PPA

A patient gradually loses understanding of some words.

They may not recognize everyday objects or faces of familiar people.

Agrammatic PPA

Increased speaking difficulties

They may leave out words that link verbs and nouns (such as from, with, and to).

Gradual, complete loss of speech

Gradual movement difficulties

Logopenic PPA

Patients may experience difficulties choosing the right words during conversations despite understanding sentences and phrases.

They may have trouble expressing ideas despite retaining good grammar skills.

Frontotemporal dementia does not have designated tests that one can just carry out to determine whether they have it. Doctors order usual tests and conduct physical examinations to rule out conditions with similar symptoms and signs to diagnose properly. If necessary, they then assess the patient's reflexes, muscle strength, and other important functions. The healthcare providers also test the patient's problem-solving, attention, and counting skills to determine the level of cognitive damage, if any. Doctors then order a computed tomography (CT) scan, or magnetic resonance imaging (MRI) to locate the damaged areas and assess, in real-time, the level of damage made to the brain.

There is currently no cure for frontotemporal dementia, but healthcare professionals prescribe medication to treat symptoms. Patients may use antidepressant and antipsychotic medications to treat anxiety and fight compulsive behaviors.

Vascular Dementia

Also called Multi-Infarct Dementia, Vascular Dementia refers to a decline in cognition skills due to reduced or blocked blood supply to the brain, causing oxygen and nutrient deprivation and, eventually, death of the brain cells.

Patients with vascular dementia experience different symptoms depending on the location and severity of blood flow impairment in the brain. Symptoms of vascular dementia can be sudden, or they may develop gradually, progressing over time. They may also overlap with other dementia forms, such as Alzheimer's disease. However, unlike Alzheimer's disease, patients with vascular dementia often show symptoms that involve difficulties in problem-solving and changes in the speed of thought, rather than loss of memory. When symptoms follow a recent stroke and clearly seem related, the condition may be referred to as post-stroke dementia.

Vascular dementia patients may experience:

- challenges in paying attention to details or concentrating on the same activity for a long time
- depression
- a decline in the ability to organize actions or thoughts
- agitation and restlessness
- reduced ability to plan and communicate ideas or logically analyze situations
- confusion
- reduced thinking speed
- apathy
- unsteady gait
- reduced or complete loss of bladder control

Doctors perform neurocognitive tests to evaluate the patient's judgment, planning, memory, and other cognitive skills. When healthcare providers scan and test patients, they often find brain abnormalities that show proof of prior strokes, but this does not mean that every individual who has experienced a stroke will also suffer from dementia.

White matter is a system of deep neural connections that links brain lobes. In people with vascular dementia, doctors may also detect changes in the white matter.

Symptoms of vascular dementia are manageable with the proper medications. Doctors may prescribe drugs that prevent stroke to reduce the chances of additional damage to the brain. Lifestyle changes also help reduce the risk of getting related health complications. These good health practices include weight management, watching alcohol consumption, and staying away from cigarettes.

Mixed Dementia

In some instances, a patient may exhibit signs of more than one form of dementia, called Mixed Dementia. Symptoms of mixed dementia differ based on the affected brain regions, forms of dementia involved, and severity of damage to the brain.

Other Conditions

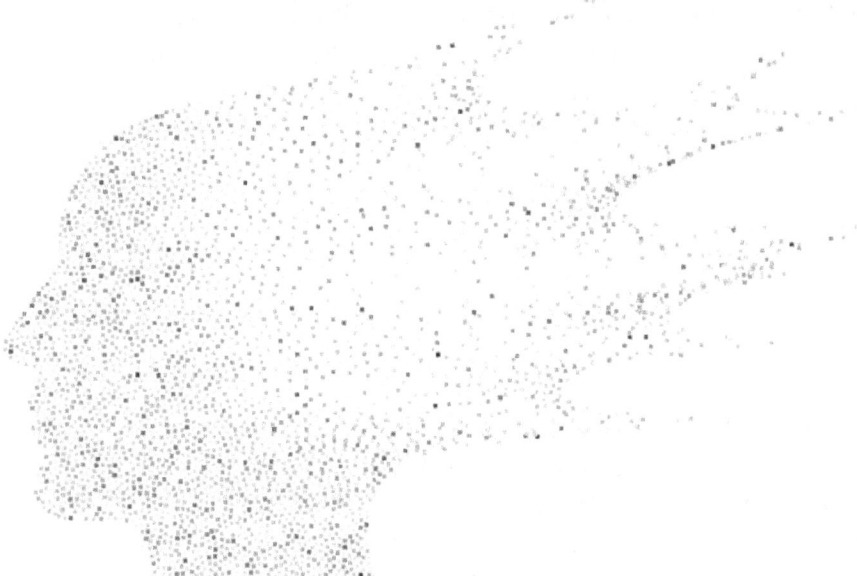

Apart from the neurological diseases discussed above, various conditions cause dementia in patients. Because some conditions shield themselves behind illnesses with similar symptoms, you must learn about other conditions that cause dementia and how they occur.

Creutzfeldt-Jakob Disease

A malformation of proteins called prions causes other prion proteins in the brain to misfold, giving rise to rare neurodegenerative diseases known as prion diseases. Creutzfeldt-Jakob disease (CJD) is the most common form of prion disease in humans and causes dementia. Unlike many other forms of dementia, CJD causes dementia that progresses fast. Malformed prion proteins destroy brain cells, causing an unusually rapid decline in cognitive function. The disease is generally classified into the following types.

Sporadic Creutzfeldt-Jakob Disease

Spontaneously develops, usually between 60 and 65 years of age.

Familial Creutzfeldt-Jakob Disease

Stems from chromosomal changes in the biological makeup of prion protein.

Develops in individuals who would have genetically inherited the chromosomal abnormalities.

Manifests in individuals at a younger age than the sporadic Creutzfeldt-Jakob disease.

Acquired Creutzfeldt-Jakob Disease

This disease is caused by external exposure to abnormal prion protein resulting from some medical procedures or food infected with bovine spongiform encephalopathy, a neurodegenerative disorder in cattle.

Symptoms

As with the discussed forms of dementia, different people with Creutzfeldt-Jakob disease may experience various symptoms, and the severity differs from each individual. At some point in the progression of the disease, patients with this disease experience:

- disorientation
- muscle stiffness, twitches, and involuntary jerky movements
- confusion and depression
- indifference, irritability, and mood swings
- hallucinations or double vision

- walking difficulties
- memory loss and poor judgment

Diagnosis

Like most other conditions that cause dementia, there is no designated test to precisely diagnose Creutzfeldt-Jakob disease in living humans. Still, a series of tests can help reveal if a person is *likely* to develop Creutzfeldt-Jakob disease.

- Electroencephalogram (EEG) measures electrical activity at the brain level and shows the patterns
- Brain magnetic resonance imaging (MRI) detects specific brain abnormalities related to Creutzfeldt-Jakob disease
- Lumbar puncture (spinal tap) checks for particular proteins in the spinal fluid
- Protein misfolding cyclic amplification (PMCA) detects malformed protein aggregates

Huntington's Disease

Another disease that causes dementia in patients is Huntington's disease (HD). It is a progressive disorder of the brain caused by a defective gene. When it strikes, it affects the central nervous system, causing challenges in thinking, moving, and social interaction. Individuals born to families with a history of HD and who inherit the defective gene eventually develop Huntington's disease.

Symptoms

Huntington's disease usually manifests between ages 30 and 50, although symptoms can still appear earlier or later. The main sign of the disease is loss of movement control in the arms, legs, and upper body. It also affects reasoning, memory, judgment, and plan execution. Patients with HD eventually struggle with depression, anxiety, and irritability.

Diagnosis

Individuals eager to know if they have HD can take a genetic test to determine whether they carry the defective gene, even if they do not have any outward symptoms.

Normal Pressure Hydrocephalus (NPH)

In some unfortunate cases, excess cerebrospinal fluid pools in some parts of the brain, causing a brain disorder called normal pressure hydrocephalus. The fluid buildup could stem from tumors, infection, head injuries, or hemorrhaging. Due to the excess cerebrospinal fluid, brain ventricles enlarge to the extent that disturbs and damages the surrounding brain tissue. The disorder impairs one's thought processes and physical abilities. NPH gets its name because measured cerebrospinal fluid pressure usually remains normal despite the extra fluid.

Specialists can treat normal pressure by surgically inserting a shunt to drain the excess fluid from the brain. A successful surgery resolves walking challenges, but thought processes usually remain an issue.

Symptoms

Individuals with normal pressure hydrocephalus may show:

- walking difficulties
- mild dementia
- loss of bladder control

Diagnosis

Healthcare providers perform the following tests to confirm whether a patient has normal pressure hydrocephalus. Depending on the patient's presentation and other factors, they may carry out one or more tests.

Brain imaging

Specialists use a computed tomography scan or magnetic resonance imaging to detect changes in the brain ventricles.

Clinical examination

Neurologists clinically examine patients with suspected normal pressure hydrocephalus to evaluate the damage and rule out other conditions like Alzheimer's.

Cerebrospinal Fluid Tests

The following tests are also crucial as they are used to estimate shunt responsiveness:

- lumbar puncture
- external lumbar drainage
- cerebrospinal fluid outflow resistance
- intracranial pressure monitoring
- isotope cisternography

Korsakoff Syndrome

Vitamin B, also called thiamin, helps maintain brain function by facilitating energy production. Brain cells fail to produce enough energy to support brain processes without enough thiamin. Severe thiamine deficiency disturbs the processing of brain signals and affects the storage and retrieval of memories. When thiamine deficiency interferes with normal brain functioning, brain cells suffer significant damage accompanied by microscopic bleeding. Damage resulting from the considerable thiamin crisis causes a central nervous system disorder called Korsakoff syndrome. The condition also results from various other causes ranging from serious health issues such as advanced cancers to something as simple as poor food choices. Korsakoff syndrome can also occur in individuals who struggle with proper food absorption or alcohol misuse.

Korsakoff syndrome often follows another neurological syndrome called Wernicke encephalopathy (WE). Wernicke Encephalopathy is a life-threatening emergency characterized by fatal brain disruption, abnormal eye movements, and lack of coordination. Although WE usually precedes Korsakoff syndrome, individuals without prior WE history can still develop Korsakoff syndrome.

Symptoms

Despite most patients being able to hold conversations and socialize as normal, they may encounter:

- trouble retaining new information
- long-term memory gaps
- difficulties remembering recent events
- hallucinations

In many cases, the patients may unintentionally fabricate the lost information to fill in the blanks in memory.

It is sometimes challenging to diagnose Korsakoff syndrome as its symptoms may hide behind other health problems such as head injuries and alcohol intoxication. Since there are no specific imaging or laboratory tests to determine if an individual has Korsakoff syndrome, the job lies in the hands of a specialized healthcare provider.

Alzheimer's Disease

And finally, Alzheimer's disease. Alzheimer's disease is an irreversible neurological disease that disrupts normal brain function, altering one's behavior, memory, and thought processes.

Stages of Alzheimer's Disease

Alzheimer's disease develops slowly, worsening gradually over the years. As time goes on, the condition eventually disturbs most areas of the brain, such as those controlling language, judgment, and other cognitive functions.

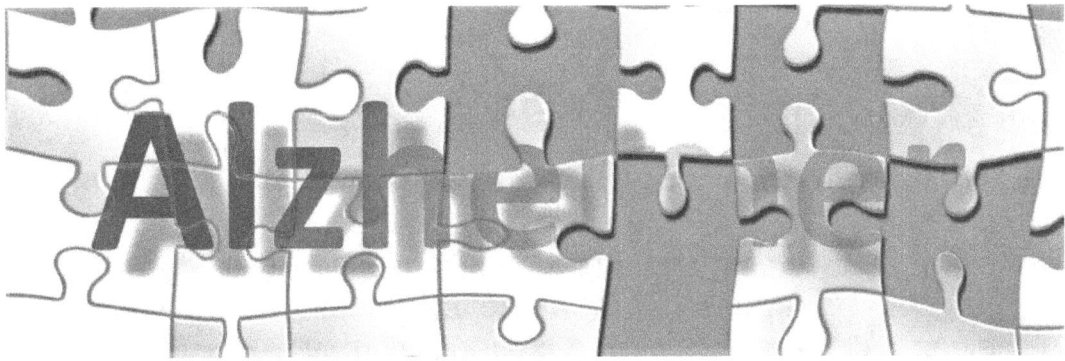

When researching, you may find it classified into three or seven stages, but we will discuss five. Although this book focuses on the early stages of the disease, learning and understanding other stages is an integral part of your caregiving journey. By learning how the stages vary and progress, you understand the changes that await your LO and can prepare to the best of your capacity. Alzheimer's disease progresses continuously, so you should realize that the discussed stages are only for reference and comprehension.

Stage 1

Alzheimer's disease is so cunning that it develops subtly, causing minor brain changes that can go unnoticed for years. In research settings, the early signs can be identified before symptoms manifest. This stage of normal outward behavior is called the preclinical phase. Neither the patient nor the caregiver notices signs of Alzheimer's disease during the preclinical stage, and the patient can remain in this stage for years.

Only special imaging tests can show whether one has the disease during this stage. With the current advancements in technology, it is possible to identify deposits of the characteristic feature of Alzheimer's disease, a protein called amyloid-beta, using advanced imaging techniques. With a doctor's recommendation, some individuals seek genetic testing to determine their risk of developing Alzheimer's disease.

Stage 2

The changes in behavior at this stage are very minimal, and you might still miss them. Patients in this phase may misplace minor items or forget words they do not usually use, which is why changes at this stage are difficult to address. People at this stage of Alzheimer's disease continue to live and work as expected, without needing extra help with simple activities.

Later during this phase, patients develop mild cognitive impairment, causing mild but noticeable changes in their thinking and memory.

They may experience memory lapses regarding simple information, such as recent events, appointments, or conversations. Patients at this stage may also have challenges judging the amount of time needed to complete tasks, and others may find it hard to make proper decisions.

Stage 3

During the third stage of Alzheimer's disease, your LO shows clear, unmistakable signs of cognitive decline. Healthcare professionals diagnose most patients at this stage when caregivers or family members worry about the symptoms interfering with their LO's daily activities. The patient may forget the names of new people just after meeting them, repeat the same questions you have already answered, or may display more difficulties in planning tasks.

Stage 4

Patients grow more forgetful and confused by the time they reach this stage. They may occasionally lose track of location and time and show difficulties remembering their phone number, address, or other personal details. It also becomes a challenge to choose appropriate clothes for different events, so they may need extra help to complete daily tasks and care for themselves.

Stage 5

In the advanced phases of Alzheimer's disease, your LO may forget people's names, faces, or both. As the damage progresses, patients mistake familiar people for others. Delusions eventually kick in with the progression of this stage, and your LO might think they should go to work or visit a particular friend. In reality, however, they may not have a job, or the friend in question could be deceased. This is a difficult phase as your LO may need help with sensitive tasks such as using the bathroom and dressing up.

Later during this stage, your LO undergoes severe cognitive decline and loses basic abilities such as eating, sitting up, or walking. This is when they need genuine, extensive care the most because they may even lose the ability to tell when they are hungry or thirsty.

Although challenging, many families resort to special facilities such as nursing homes or memory care centers when they realize they cannot provide as much care and attention as their LO needs.

Symptoms of Alzheimer's Disease

The disease manifests differently in different stages and people. Symptoms may vary from occasional anxiety to loss of impulse control and even seizures. It is an essential part of positive caregiving to learn more about these signs as it helps determine how fast or slow the disease is progressing. When you know the rate at which the disease develops, you can appropriately adjust the amount of attention you give the patient. Let's take a look at some of the symptoms:

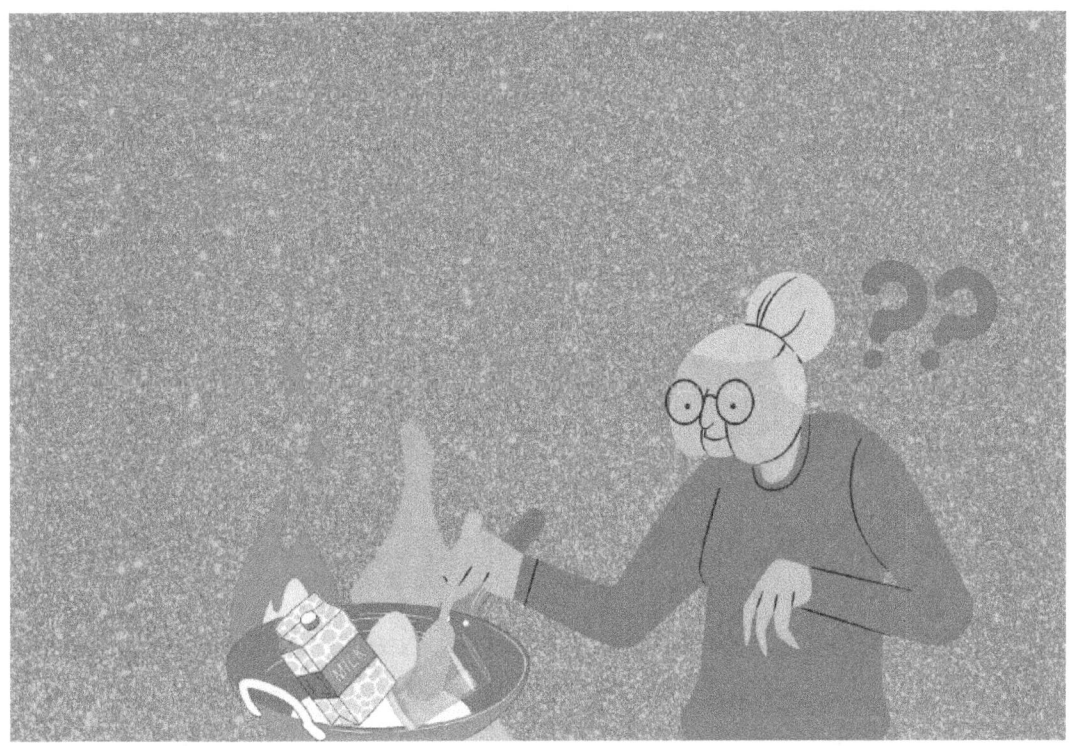

Early-onset Alzheimer's Disease

- Visual processing challenges
- They may have trouble understanding or estimating distance.
- They may encounter difficulties reading things that they once could read without problems.
- Forgetfulness
- They may mistake days of the week and lose track of dates.
- They may lose track of recent conversations.
- They may forget where they put essential items.
- Poor judgment

- They may encounter challenges in handling financial matters.
- They may find it overwhelming to follow instructions such as recipe methods.
- Loss of independence or control
- Physical problems

They may have difficulties in:
- Walking
- Speaking
- Swallowing
- Decreased expression
- Patients may have challenges describing objects.
- They may have difficulties recalling words they once knew.
- They may have trouble putting ideas into words.
- Getting lost
- Patients may leave the house and forget where they want to go.
- They may have trouble finding their way in once-familiar places.
- Personality changes

Now that we have explored dementia and covered the basics of Alzheimer's disease, we will dissect caregiving elements in the chapters ahead, one after the other.

Chapter 2:

What Is Caregiving?

I never wanted to be a burden to my kids. I don't want them to feel they HAVE to do everything for me. I can still do things for myself

—Mom

A caregiver assists and supports someone with daily activities such as grooming, housekeeping, and personal affairs management. But an Alzheimer's caregiver offers so much more than that: Proper caregiving provides your LO with support and companionship that significantly helps manage the progression of the disease. We'll discuss how to take care of your LO from the point they get diagnosed.

You may need a team for support during your caregiving journey, and the good news is This Book wants in on your team so you will never be alone. In this chapter, we will explore the many facets of caregiving. First, let's talk about the first phase of your journey—the diagnosis.

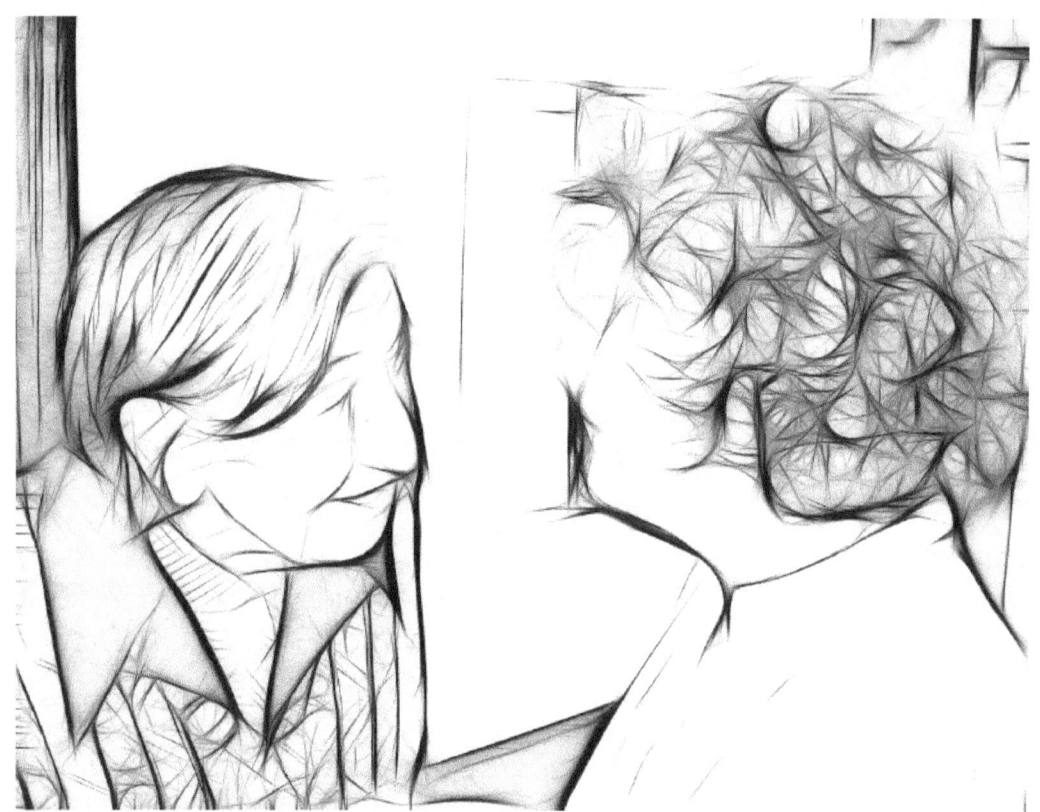

The diagnosis of Alzheimer's is hard to accept and deal with, but getting the news early in life can be disruptive and disheartening. It often settles like a huge dark cloud, threatening to dim all the light one has ever known. The diagnosis is as disturbing to your LO as it is to you, so you have to team up and go through it together. While some people just take the news as it is and move on, it could take others time to come to terms with the life-altering news. Whether you take it head-on or need time to mule over it, that is okay because we all process matters differently. Don't take months to come around because this is hard on your LO, too!

In some cases, your LO may hide their diagnosis from you. When they finally muster the courage to share, understand that they may have had reasons not to do so earlier. Sometimes people hide important issues from us because they think it is to protect us;

maybe your LO did not want to bother you during your final months on an important project, or they were in denial and needed time to take it in. Instead of overreacting and overthinking, appreciate them opening up in the end.

Alzheimer's disease occurs even in people who take the utmost care of themselves by eating healthy food, exercising, and visiting their doctors often. Even though it is not your LO's fault to get a diagnosis, they could repeatedly question themself, trying to figure out what they did wrong. If they need more time to process their own feelings; be it sadness, despair, or anger; and bid their old life goodbye, please let them. It is vital that they freely process everything because that helps them define what steps they will take to move on. Allowing your LO time to grieve lets you clear your mind as you prepare for the journey ahead.

Some LOs underestimate their relevance and may even engage in self-pity, thinking the diagnosis changes how their families and friends see them, but that is not the case—at least it should not be. Despite the life-changing diagnosis, your LO is still the same person they were days before finding out; they remain your family or friend, and they still matter. Anyone who has conducted enough research would agree their LO still has a lot of life to enjoy and that being diagnosed with early-onset Alzheimer's disease is not the end. Several daring caregivers successfully mark this point as only the beginning of a new adventure. Letting your LO know they still have a purpose warms their heart and encourages them to cooperate so they do not lose hope.

During the first few days after the diagnosis, some of our LOs may find it challenging to discuss their thoughts, not as an effect of the disease but as a psychological response to the discovery. If your LO cannot open up to you, encourage them to talk to someone—anyone with whom they feel comfortable; a doctor, therapist, or close friend. Sharing thoughts and emotions enables other concerned parties to assist your LO in coping with the diagnosis and open up to you. Recommending them to talk to someone trustworthy despite not wanting to share with you shows them that you want the best for them and are only trying to support them. With time, they will acknowledge your support and cooperate.

Caregiving Responsibilities

Whether you hire a professional caregiver to assist you in taking care of your LO or decide to take on most of the work yourself, understanding the job description is essential because it helps you prepare and adjust accordingly.

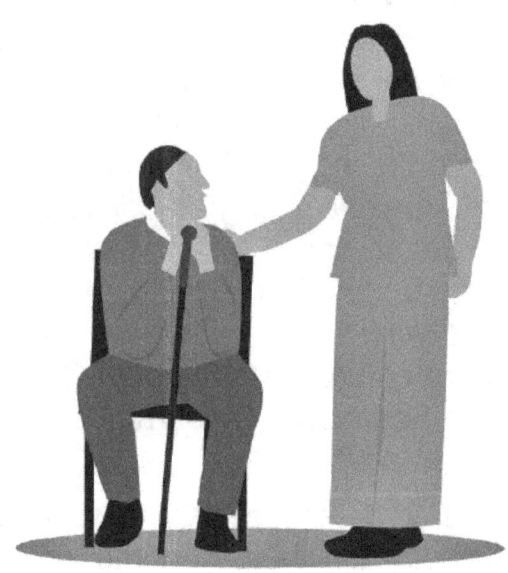

Develop understanding

It would help your caregiving journey if you were to devote part of your precious time to learning the effect of the disease on your LO and on you. You cannot tackle and survive caregiving if you do not understand what it demands of you and what your LO is going through. When you develop awareness, you have a better chance of nailing the expectations.

Offer basic support

While your LO may still be able to carry out most tasks independently, please assist them with tasks they find challenging. If you notice inconsistencies in the functions they need extra help with, that could be a sign their range of abilities is deteriorating. Although they may already have trouble concentrating, another way to support them is to keep them engaged and entertained. You can read stories, watch their favorite shows, or do any other activities they would be interested in. This helps them feel loved and relaxed.

Provide emotional support

Genuine emotional support has a positive influence on your LO. They need to feel understood, and if you do this right, your LO will notice the difference and learn to trust you more. When they feel excluded by society, be their emotional pillar and help them through it because heightened stress levels have a negative impact on their health and may fuel the progression of the disease. Knowing they have you for a friend gives them security, helps aggravate their worries and gives them strength to carry on fighting.

Monitor them closely

Because some activities may trigger anxiety, or your LO may lose interest in activities they once enjoyed, you can help ensure they do everything they are supposed to do to make them comfortable. Although some of our LOs with early-onset Alzheimer's disease may still be able to whip up tasty meals, others may find cooking overwhelming. Consider monitoring their diet and ensuring your LO gets all the nutrients they need in sufficient quantities. Financial issues are another hurdle you should be prepared to take care of. Dealing with finances, legal matters, and even technologies such as spam calls and emails could be infuriating for your LO, but that is where you come in to save the day. In a later chapter, we'll discuss strategies for aiding your LO with these matters.

Caregiving Strategies

You may find yourself confronted by various mixed emotions during your caregiving journey. Sometimes you could be driven by genuine empathy and concern, while other times, you are overwhelmed by anxiety and frustration.

Although you may feel obliged to put your LO's needs above yours, the caregiving role requires that you take care of yourself first. Consider your last trip by air and the flight attendant instructing you to put your own oxygen mask on before assisting others. This same principle applies to caregiving. Your reasons for putting your LO first probably make sense to you; otherwise, you wouldn't do it, but the reason you should practice self-care is simple. We will discuss some specific self-care strategies you can implement in a later chapter.

Exercise patience

People with Alzheimer's disease may take a little longer than usual to process questions, so indirect questions, instructions, or remarks only cause confusion that can otherwise be avoided. Because they also tend to ask some questions repeatedly, you must try your best to respond calmly, without a blatant display of frustration. To optimize their understanding, simplify your instructions, questions, and feedback with clear communication.

Due to the slight changes in their thinking processes, your LO may need more time to complete tasks than the average individual. While it could sound like a good idea to do the tasks on your own instead of waiting ages for your LO to complete their tasks, taking on their responsibilities is not advisable. Firstly, it takes away their sense of purpose, confirming their fear that they may be irrelevant or incompetent, or worse, giving them the impression you are taking away their control over their lives. Stripping their duties off their shoulders also discourages LOs from trying other tasks because you would have planted it into their minds that what they do carries only nominal value.

Instead of turning down their help completely or doing everything for them, involve them in simple tasks that they can still carry out without much difficulty. Another way to help your LO as you practice patience in caregiving is by providing choices. Some people in the early stages of the disease may already have difficulties making decisions independently. You could help them by suggesting options such as asking if they want to eat beef or chicken; instead of asking them open-ended questions such as what they want to eat.

Schedule wisely

Managing a life for two, your workload also compounds, and you may find yourself torn between your personal life and caregiving duties. One sure way to combat this before you burn out is by creating a solid routine. A practical schedule helps you strike a balance in your life, reinforcing familiarity with your LO. For example, they should know what time to bathe and what follows after bathing because the consistency helps them prepare for their tasks in advance. Create a manageable routine you and your LO can follow without feeling restricted. Your schedule allows for minor changes to accommodate times when your LO acts a little out of the usual. Avoid significant modifications to the routine because abrupt changes can confuse or even leave them less willing to cooperate.

Schedules are not only limited to tasks in and around the house, but you can also compile all outside engagements that your LO might have and sort them by time. These include doctor's visits, social engagements, and even business appointments. Taking note of these important dates significantly lightens your role and makes you efficient, ensuring your LO attends all their important appointments.

Promote a healthy diet

Some of our LOs lose track of mealtimes, forget to cook, or even eat twice the amount due to not remembering previous meals in the early stages of the disease. You can help them plan a proper diet and ensure they eat nutritious meals on time each day. It is also helpful to make the food appetizing before serving, encouraging them to eat more. Because people with Alzheimer's disease quickly lose focus, remove distractions during mealtimes and ensure their only task is cleaning their plate. Where a standard diet falls short, fill up the gap with dietary supplements such as special nutritious shakes and multivitamins. Of course, be sure to validate any changes to your LO's diet with a nutrition specialist.

Provide a comfortable environment

Find ways to make your LO comfortable while maintaining safety. Since some of them tend to feel uncomfortable in strange places or with new people, it is a good idea that you stay on the lookout for signs of disinterest and suggest a different activity that they may enjoy. If your LO still drives, lookout for any inconsistencies that could end up causing accidents. If you find a concerning issue about their driving, talk to them about letting you help but be careful to do so without making them feel uncomfortable. Make them understand that you only want to ensure their safety, not take away their freedom.

Sometimes, our LOs can feel as though their lives ended when they received their diagnosis, and they just want out of their body because sometimes it betrays them so much that they are confident it is no longer theirs. You and I both know they are still the same person, albeit with new challenges, so you would do well to help them feel comfortable just being themselves. Take steps to improve their personal hygiene, ensuring they bathe and dress well. If your LO used to wear makeup, there is no need to stop now. Help them pick the best shades and genuinely compliment them.

Another consideration, especially in later stages, is that taking care of a pet brings your LO joy in so many ways; the mutual love, lack of judgment, and a sense of being there for someone or something dependent on them for their care. Please consider this a healthy option when discussing their pet's long-term care strategy. If your LO already has a pet, taking care of it on their own may become challenging with time. They could forget to feed or bathe it, and you would have to put your expert caregiving tips to use. If you are not comfortable with animal companions, try and see the positive impact that the pet has on your LO. Understanding that the pet makes your role more manageable by keeping them company in your absence can help you rethink your perspective. However, if pets still do not sit well with you, discuss available options with your LO.

Seek help

Should you need extra advice or assistance, do not hesitate to seek help. You need different groups of people for help with different classes of issues. Ask for help from community members when you have challenges that the community can help with, and seek more comprehensive support if you need expert advice from reliable professionals.

Caregiving Don'ts

Don't interrogate them

Several caregivers admit having quizzed their LOs more than once before learning that it offers no benefit. You may want to ask their name, age, if they remember you, or other questions, but try to refrain from doing this as it makes them more anxious.

Don't dwell on their shortcomings

It can be quite confusing from the loss of employment to reduced concentration levels. If your LO leaves their job due to focus and concentration issues, it could lead to negative feelings, self-doubt, feelings of inadequacies, or even anger. Focusing too much on what your LO has lost and what they cannot do may worsen your relationship. Instead, emphasize their abilities and focus on what they still have because this gives them the strength to carry on.

Don't ignore them

Interact with your LO and avoid talking about them as if they were not there. Although their mind may not function as expected, they can still sense when or where they are unwanted. In some instances, individuals in the early stages of Alzheimer's can call their caregiver and forget what they want to say. It is infuriating; I agree, but ignoring them does not make it stop; it even affects your LO more.

Family members may inadvertently dismiss or ignore the diagnosed individual when they visit. They may direct questions about your LO's well-being to you. While the family could only be checking on your LO, talking about them as if they were not there makes them uncomfortable and can even disturb them mentally. If someone visits and communicates this way, subtly signal the visitor that you can discuss it later.

Don't assume they are always confused

Realize that your LO is not always out of themself. In fact, people in the early stages of the disease do not fade out as much as those in severe stages or with other forms of dementia, so do not discount everything your LO says.

They could tell you that someone left you a message and recall the entire message, but considering their condition, you could dismiss it, thinking they were confused while, in actuality, they still remembered. Many caregivers miss out on important things because they discount information from their LOs. It doesn't hurt to just thank them for letting you know, then confirm the information to be sure.

Now that we have established what Alzheimer's disease is and your role as a caregiver, I want you to take a deep breath and give yourself some grace. No one is perfect on this journey, and every path differs. Know that you are a wonderful, compassionate person with a lot of love and patience to share with your LO.

Blame it on, Grandma; I just can't help cleaning. I enjoy having my own place, so I don't burden my kids.

—Mom

A Day in Our Life	
Time	**Activity**
6 a.m.	Mom awakens. During this time, she is by herself. Even if I'm awake and lying in bed, this is a good time for me to get centered and prepare for the day ahead with a little alone time.
7 a.m.	I get up and officially start my day. Mom performs self-care, makes tea, coffee, or fills her water bottle.
10 a.m.	By now, mom's pill minder has alerted her to her first dose of medication for the day. I usually visit Mom and confirm she's taken her morning medication. Mom engages in her usual cleaning routine. Consistency is my mom's best friend. Regardless of how clean I find her apartment, she takes joy in the calming and repetitive nature of her routine.
11 a.m.	Mom sits down for her first meal of the day. She sometimes makes herself a delightful plate of eggs cooked anyway and a piece of fruit. We'll take this time to determine if groceries are needed several times a week and subsequently place a delivery order. I

	love grocery delivery because whether I'm home and can't get away from the computer or somewhere else, I can ensure she gets what she needs without going to the grocery store.
1 p.m.	Mom enjoys streaming her movies or may treat herself to a trip to the library or her favorite dollar store. She says the trip is to get "staples for her pantry," but I know it's to get the occasional treat.
3 p.m.	Mom delivers mail or packages to me upstairs. I'll pull up the doorbell camera and watch for any falls or lockouts when I hear the doorbell. I usually see her engaging with the postal service person or UPS driver with a smile and well wish.
5 p.m.	Dinner time! Sometimes I cook dinner, she makes something, or we'll even cook together. I also use this time to make sure she takes her evening medication.
7 p.m.	Mom retires for the evening, usually with a hug but always with a warm sentiment such as, "Sweet Dreams, baby girl" or an "I love you." And the cycle repeats the next day!

Story Time – It Begins

My caregiving journey started around 2018 when Mom living with me made good financial sense. Later, I moved to Chicago to explore a new job opportunity, city, and overall, experience a new chapter in my life, but Mom felt lonely and exhibited symptoms of depression. I asked if she wanted to move to Chicago to address her concern, and she agreed. We rented multiple-bedroom apartments from that point so that she could have her own space. Living together in this capacity, I first noticed signs of forgetfulness and repeating herself. She also expressed frustration with remembering clients' names or using computer systems at work.

One day, Mom called me in tears as she'd started a new, less stressful job at a local grocery store. The person she was paired with for training was younger and worked at a faster pace. My mom broke down, feeling awful that she couldn't keep up with remembering the grocery codes used to ring up purchases. I went to her immediately, picked her up, parked, and spent hours just letting her vent her frustrations. There were a lot of tears and hugs that day; just the two of us, a single car in a massive parking lot. That was the tipping point, and we jointly decided to pursue her permanent retirement.

Later that year, I bought a multi-unit building where Mom and I shared one of the units. Not long after, I realized I had the tenant from hell living in the other unit! Mom and I bumped heads while sharing the same space until I hatched a plan to let her have the

> other apartment. It was an excellent solution we both loved because now I have peace of mind knowing the apartment is in good hands, she can still have her independence, and there was nothing but a staircase separating us in case of an emergency. Although I still worry about her when I am away, she puts in the effort to manage most situations independently.

Prepare for some changes in your relationship. Helping your LO make important decisions can feel like you are just deciding for them, and if these are decisions that they used to make on their own, the role reversal can feel strange. In my case, Mom gave me deference and started consulting with me in an almost permission-seeking demeanor. The roles were reversed, and I hated it, lol. Finding a balance between helping my mom maintain her independence and "granting her permission" was the weirdest conundrum I had ever experienced. Sounds familiar? If your LO used to manage their finances and other important legal or medical matters, then the considerable responsibility suddenly falling into your lap, handling the problems, can be overwhelming.

You may also realize changes in your relationships with friends and other family members. Some people tend to keep their distance when they don't know what to say or how they can help. In most cases, giving you space is their way of helping. Have you experienced something like this? How did you handle it? The central question is: Can you do this by yourself?

Story Time – Better Together

> In my case, there wasn't really a second thought at first because Mom was still Mom, just occasionally repeating herself. That was before the global

> pandemic presented itself, challenging me to work from home. I had to spend more time with mom and had no outside social stimulation. I internalized a small degree of guilt for showing my frustration with her disease and was not communicating well enough with my brothers. This pressure and shame further led to self-isolation, feelings of dread, and hopelessness because they all pooled in me, but I had no outlet. With time, I sought help from a mental health coach who helped me process my normal feelings and encouraged me to approach my family for help. I am glad I did because offers came flooding in.

I cannot imagine how my situation would have worsened had I not received external help. I would go so far as to say I was spiraling into potentially dangerous territory. I could not have done it alone, and you shouldn't have to go through this by yourself, which brings me to: *building a team*.

In the next chapter, we will explore the various advantages of a support team on your caregiving journey and how to build the best support team for your LO.

Chapter 3:

Building Your Support Team

I love our doctor and my dedicated medical care team. I get a little anxious when we have to see a different doctor every time for every little thing.

—Mom

The numerous things we can say about caregiving do not change; it is exhausting and can leave even the most enduring people overwhelmed and alone. You sign up for years of evolving responsibilities when starting your caregiving journey. The most resilient caregivers forge their way through the first few months or years, comforting themselves with the idea that their LO is still the same person—which is true, but in a different way. With time, they realize they gave too much of themselves to fulfilling their obligations as caregivers, and that is when negative feelings and thoughts surge through their veins and mind, threatening to leave them sad, alone, and disheartened.

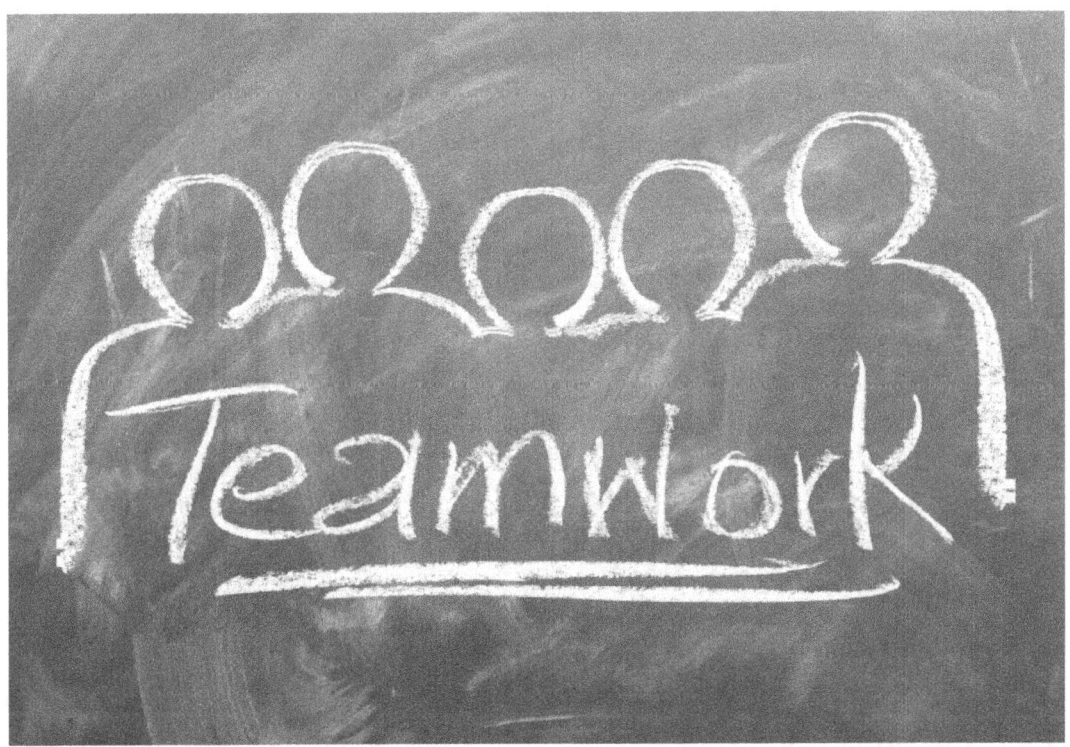

It is vital that you know the signs of stress in caregiving because burnout is real. When you understand how the road feels when the journey is about to get stormy with its twists and turns, you'll know when to slow down and let the storm pass.

The emotional and mental stress that remains uncontrolled over a long time is harmful to your health as a caregiver and has a generous amount of adverse effects on your LO. Here are some common signs of caregiver stress to watch out for:

- frequent headaches
- exhaustion
- constant sadness or feelings of emptiness
- uncharacteristic anger
- alcohol and drug abuse, including prescription drugs

- persistent body pain and unusual sleep patterns
- constant anxiety
- loss of interest in activities you once enjoyed
- little to no social interaction
- significant weight loss or gain

Have you experienced some of the symptoms above? If you have, it could be a sign that the demands of caregiving are taking a toll on your well-being. If you are experiencing some of these signs, please seek medical attention. Otherwise, continue reading for helpful tips others like you and I have done to alleviate some of these stresses.

<u>Emphasize what you offer best</u>

There is no such thing as a perfect caregiver. We make mistakes and learn every day; it is all part of the process, and there is no cheating the system. While it is normal to feel that our best is not good enough, it is crucial to understand that every effort counts. Feelings of guilt are common, and we all experience them at some point down the caregiving path. What you do about those feelings is what matters. Focus on delivering the best care you can.

<u>Be practical</u>

Although several people in the early stages of the disease may not present many challenges that need you to stay up at night, caregiving is still a full-time job, and treating it as such lightens your burden. If you have a job or business to run, you may have realized that something can come up at work when your LO needs you close. Lightly assuming you can manage both simultaneously would put you under unnecessary pressure. As you set your goals and plans, consider your job or business and think everything through before taking on an unrealistic schedule as part of your routine. Spend your energy and time on problems you can solve, not on unrealistic expectations that often lead to frustration and despair.

Acknowledge your effort

You are there, and you are trying. That is what's important. Your LO recognizes the work you put in, and they are grateful even if they might not say it. Whenever you feel your effort is not enough or no one recognizes it, remember that everything you do to support your LO counts, and it does not matter if no one else seems to notice. If you still don't realize how much you are helping, keep a small notepad to track all the significant things you do in hopes of improving the life of your LO.

Above all, a sure way to avoid burnout is by accepting that you do not have to do this alone, not when you can have a team on which to rely. In the next section, find out what makes the team important for your caregiving journey.

Why Have a Support Team?

A support team is a group of reliable people who share a mutual goal: to provide support and care throughout the caregiving journey. You are still the primary caregiver within a support team, just not carrying the burden alone. Building a support team minimizes stress and your chances of getting overwhelmed. A team also gives you a necessary outlet and opportunity to enjoy your life without worrying about how your LO is faring without you.

Shared responsibility

Teamwork in caregiving simplifies the job for involved members while ensuring efficiency through labor division. When working alone, you are responsible for carrying out all the necessary tasks, and if you leave midway, you will pick tasks up from where you left them. Fortunately, your absence or outside appointments do not put caregiving tasks on hold with a support team because one of the team members with a different work schedule or skill set can cover for you. Those tasks can include shopping, cleaning, cooking, and taking your LO out for fun or even various appointments.

Improved flexibility

Having a support team on standby helps improve your quality of life by increasing flexibility in your schedule, allowing you to live your life once in a while. If you take occasional breaks when your body needs to rest, you become more productive, and your mind and body get recharged.

Information sharing

You can think about a support team as an inside hub for sharing information and exchanging skills. One team member may have extensive knowledge regarding a particular subject, while another has expertise in another area. If you choose the right people for your team, you realize there is much to learn from others around you. A dedicated group of people with different skillsets and experience in various topics is the best place to start when you have questions about your caregiving journey.

Emotional support

With a team of people who have your best interests at heart, you can share your thoughts and concerns in a relaxed manner, knowing that you are with safe company. They provide a healthy outlet for your inner self, allowing you to look deep inside yourself, digest your emotions, and outline what you could do differently the next time a challenge arises.

Social time

Let's be honest, caregiving can alienate you from the outside world because it demands a lot of time, and several caregivers sacrifice their social time. They forget that taking care of themselves is the first step to effectively caring for their LO. A support team gives you another shot at improving your social life. You can rekindle lost connections or build new friendships. Your support team is a complete package if you want to maintain a small inside circle.

Extended perspective

Some team members may have prior experience in caring for people with Alzheimer's disease, which helps maintain positive energy, reducing feelings of burnout. Experienced members help you make sense of the situation without frustrating yourself over issues beyond your control.

Steps to Build Your Support Team

Several caregivers insist on taking care of their LOs alone. People who decide to do this on their own have religious and cultural reasons. Some families do not believe in seeking outside help because they feel that it would make them appear weak or incapable. While we cannot dismiss others' traditional beliefs as misleading, the importance of teamwork in caregiving is not to be taken lightly. Other people simply feel they work better on their own because it helps them avoid conflict. Another group of people who usually refuse help are those in denial. They look at their LO and are convinced they are still there, which is valid for most people in the early stages of the disease, but extra caregiving support becomes necessary when symptoms worsen. Following are some basic strategies for building your support team from the beginning.

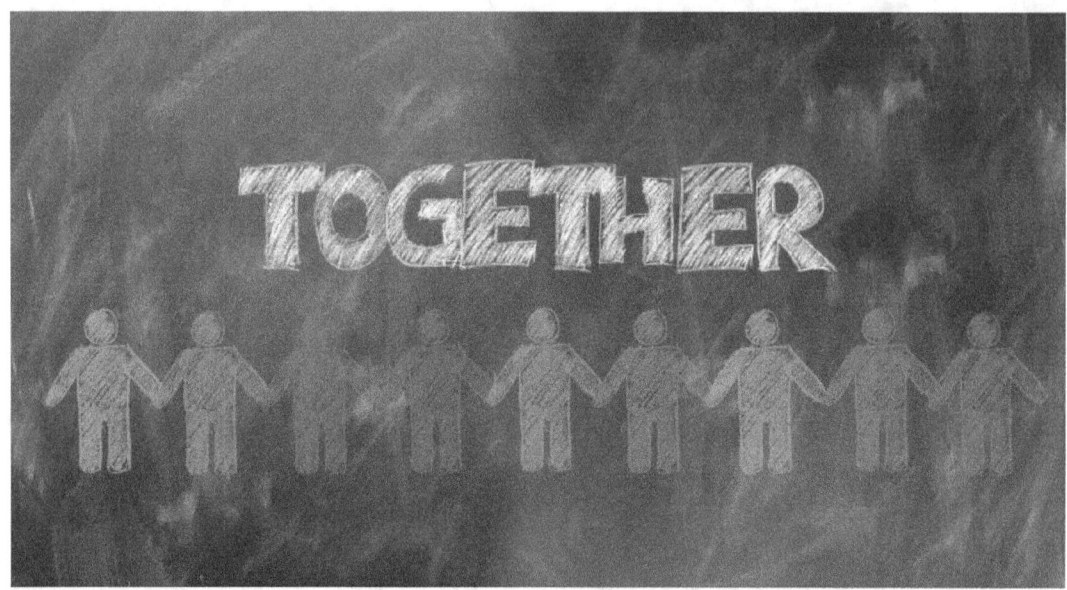

Identify the people who may be interested in helping you, and thoroughly discuss how they can help. Be transparent and sincere when asking for help, clearly stating which tasks you need help with. Avoid seeking assistance from individuals who seem judgmental as they may cause you problems in the future.

Elect ones who are compassionate, empathetic, and understanding as they will help support the cause. If someone turns you down or cannot help, understand that they could also be going through something, and appreciate their direct feedback because people who unwillingly agree to help will slow you down.

Show gratitude. Team members who feel appreciated are more likely to help you again whenever you need them. You do not have to shower your team with excessive gifts; a genuine thank you goes a long way.

Who Are They?

Your support team should include people with various skills to contribute to the team. Balance is as important when choosing a support team as planning meals. However, a combination of varied skills alone is not enough. More importantly, the team members should be reliable individuals who understand the importance of fulfilling their promises and responsibilities and respect confidentiality. Include friends, neighbors, professionals, family, and the community.

You will need someone who can help navigate eldercare to help organize the unique needs of your LO. Your support team also requires professionals well-versed in legal and financial situations to help you navigate related processes and procedures. After professional assistance comes general help around the house. You will need someone who can help with home maintenance by carrying out domestic tasks such as cleaning, cooking, etc. The individual who assists with home errands can also take your LO to the movies or meet some friends so that you can have a short break to nap, go to the spa, or interact with your friends. Even after putting together all those groups of people, your support team is incomplete without someone impartial just to listen when the road gets rough.

You can also include digital solutions and services as part of your care team for extra convenience. You can install cameras around the house to monitor falls or lockouts. Take advantage of the modern-day technological conveniences by automating home systems such as turning lights off and on, locking doors and windows, and monitoring the room's temperature. Install water sensors in the bathroom and kitchen to prevent falls. Use sensors to detect fire, smoke, gas, glass breaks, and other related hazards. You can also invest in an automated pill dispenser that locks to help your LO take their medication correctly and on time. For security purposes, you can get your LO a fashion ID bracelet that bears the contact details of someone to call in case of emergencies. You can also take a moment and visit their favorite spots, such as the library or corner store, to leave your contact information so they can reach you if your LO wanders there or something happens.

Home Safety

Your LO may be more susceptible to safety hazards in some areas in and around the house. Go ahead and evaluate their surroundings and resolve anything that could cause harm. Essential areas to pay attention to include kitchens, garages, basements, workrooms, and other places where there may be chemicals, tools, or other harmful items.

Take steps to avoid kitchen accidents. You can prevent incorrect or unsafe usage of kitchen appliances such as stoves and grinders by turning off their power supply whenever they are not in use. Keep decorative fruits, prescription drugs, and toxic plants out of reach because your LO might mistake them for food.

Keep your LO's bedroom safe and comfortable. Monitor heating pads, electric blankets, and heaters to avoid burns and injuries. Customize closet shelves to an accessible height if they are difficult to reach. The modification keeps your LO from falling while trying to reach some overhead items.

Post lists of essential emergency contacts around the house so anyone in the home can call for help in case of accidents or other emergencies. Important contacts include local fire and police departments, poison control helplines, and hospitals.

Keep rooms and pathways well-lit to avoid falls. Even the light levels in the house because inconsistent lighting can be disturbing.

Remove weapons such as guns from easily accessible places and consider locking them away to avoid disastrous misuse.

Ensure that oversized furniture items such as bookshelves and cabinets are secure to avoid tipping.

Improve bathroom safety by removing rugs and using textured stickers on slippery surfaces. You can also use grab bars for the tub and shower to provide your LO with additional support. Ensure safety in the laundry room by securing away all cleaning products to avoid possible misuse.

Lastly, vitamins or over-the-counter pain medications such as aspirin or ibuprofen, while intended to make us feel better, can be detrimental if taken in large, unmonitored quantities. It may be time to round up all of those medications that were once self-administered and keep them in a place to which only you have access.

Remember that accepting help when offered is part of the journey, even if you are the type of person who prides themselves in not needing help previously. Ask for assistance whenever the job at hand seems to be overpowering you. Understand that accepting or asking for help does NOT make you weak, nor does it mean you are not concerned about your LO. Building a support team is responsible for ensuring your LO receives quality care while your life outside caregiving continues.

Chapter 4:

Mastering Communication With Healthcare Professionals

I'm so glad you go to my doctor's appointments with me; there's no way I would have remembered all of that!
—Mom

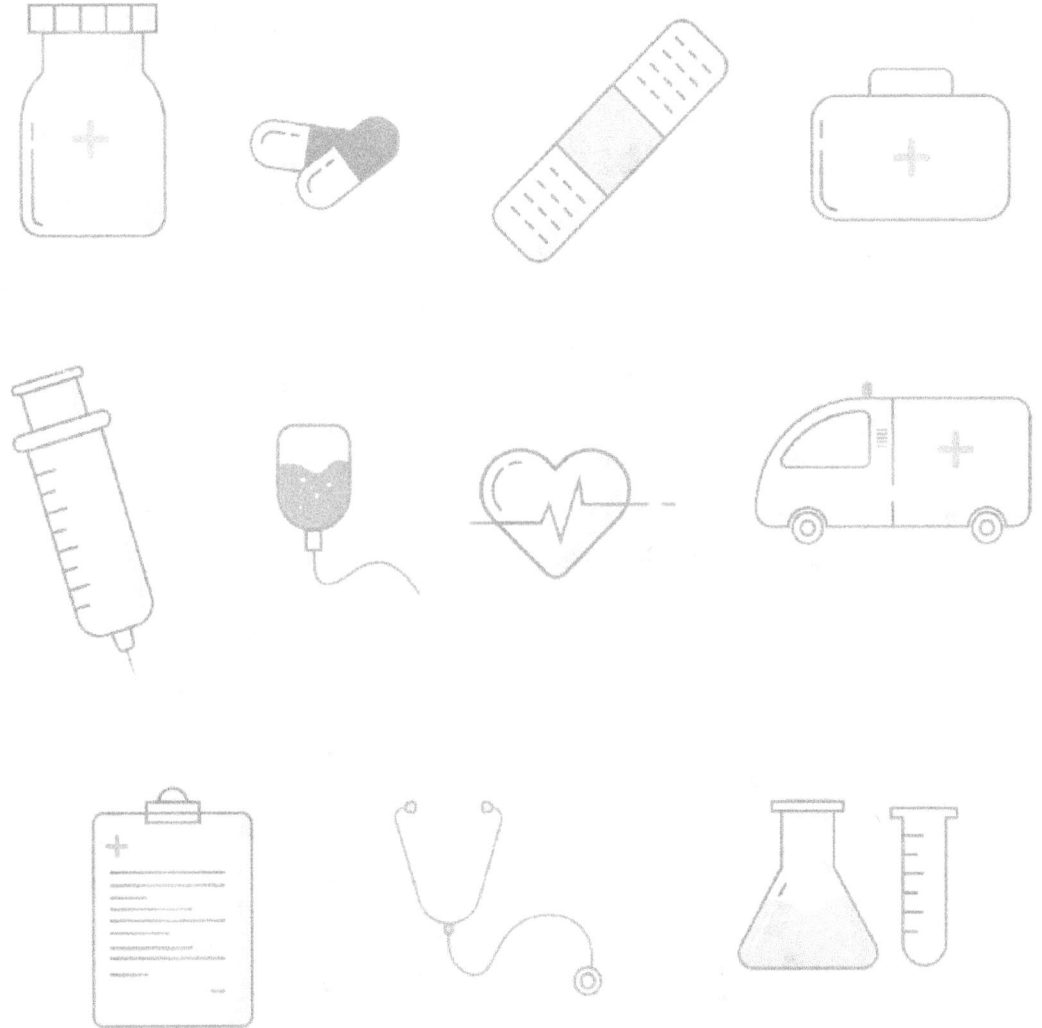

Healthcare providers are an important part of your support team, making communication with them just as critical. When caring for someone living with Alzheimer's, consider staying prepared for emergency hospital visits, as these come without warning. Emergencies can be overly stressful, but you can take steps to prepare for them as a caregiver. While the healthcare team is there to help you and your LO, how much you support them affects the quality of service they deliver. It starts with communication. Proper communication goes a long way to improve the quality of service healthcare providers deliver, so you must learn how to communicate with them.

Handling Hospital Emergencies

Hospital emergencies can be exhausting nightmares, but here are some tips to improve communication and make the experience better for you, the healthcare professionals, and your LO. Ask a flexible care team member to go with you if they are close or to meet you at the hospital. Having someone with you eases your anxiety and gives you more time to talk to healthcare providers while knowing your LO is in good company.

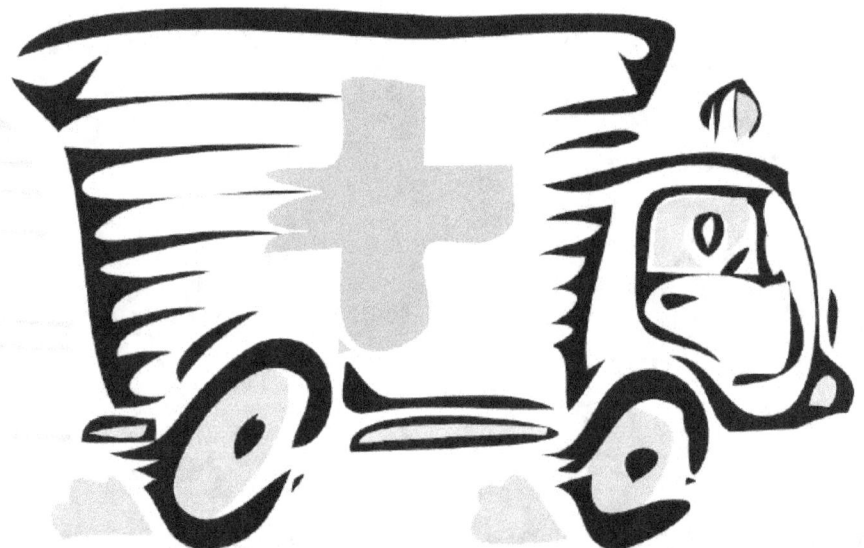

Different doctors and nurses may ask you the same questions more than once and expect you to answer them. They do not do that to annoy you but ensure they get the correct background regarding events leading to the visit. They can deduce the best way forward with details as accurate as possible.

Remind the healthcare staff that your LO has Alzheimer's disease, although they would already have the records. Give them a clear picture of the progression stage at which your LO is and explain how best to communicate with them.

Although you could be scared, try to stay calm and remain positive because your LO can absorb how you feel and become anxious. Comfort and distract them while you wait for further assistance.

Trust and respect the process. Sometimes it takes a long time for hospital staff to get back to you, but the delay is usually justifiable. Lab results could take time, and the staff cannot hurry machines, despite wanting to help as quickly as possible.

Emergency room staff may have limited training in Alzheimer's disease, so do not hesitate to give as much information as possible when prompted. That will help them better understand your LO's condition. Encourage the staff to directly address your LO as an individual, not just another patient who is disoriented.

Your LO will not always have to be admitted, but if they must remain, stay with them or ask a member of your care team to step in.

To avoid confusion and stress, keep an emergency bag ready, and make sure to include the following items:

- cash
- copies of health insurance or Medicare cards
- water and healthy snacks
- lists of treatments your LO takes, and the related conditions
- names and contact numbers of healthcare providers
- spare clothes and toiletries
- pain medicine for yourself (typically, a hospital will not allow you to administer outside medications to the admitted individual)
- a notebook to write instructions

- an extra cellphone charger

> ## Story Time – Scary Time
>
> Over the past few months, my mom and I have had a few emergency room scares that interfered with her regular routines and my work schedule and drained both of us physically and emotionally. I explained situations to the hospital staff, listed current medications and allergies, answered family history questions, and informed her doctor of mom's eating and exercise habits. I cannot stress the importance of organization enough!

Scheduled Doctor Visits

One core quality of an excellent caregiver is the ability to organize information and items for easy access in the future. The same quality is a crucial factor contributing to better communication with healthcare professionals. You can document information related to your LO's condition in a simple notebook or smartphone application. That way, you will be ready for the questions from healthcare providers during your LO's scheduled doctor visits.

<u>Track medical appointments</u>

Organize your LO's upcoming appointments together with notes from prior appointments. If healthcare providers instruct you to watch out for specific changes, document them with information regarding upcoming appointments so that you can quickly provide them to your LO's doctor when you visit.

<u>Record family history</u>

Document important notes on family history, such as the medical history of close family members. Healthcare providers often ask if other family members have had certain conditions as they narrow down what kind of help your LO needs.

<u>Document changes in daily symptoms</u>

Track your LO's daily symptoms and jot them in a logbook to track condition-related changes. In the same logbook, also record any significant changes in behavior. A logbook with daily symptoms and observed behavior changes gives your LO's healthcare team a comprehensive analysis of how the condition has progressed and helps them decide if your LO requires further tests or treatment.

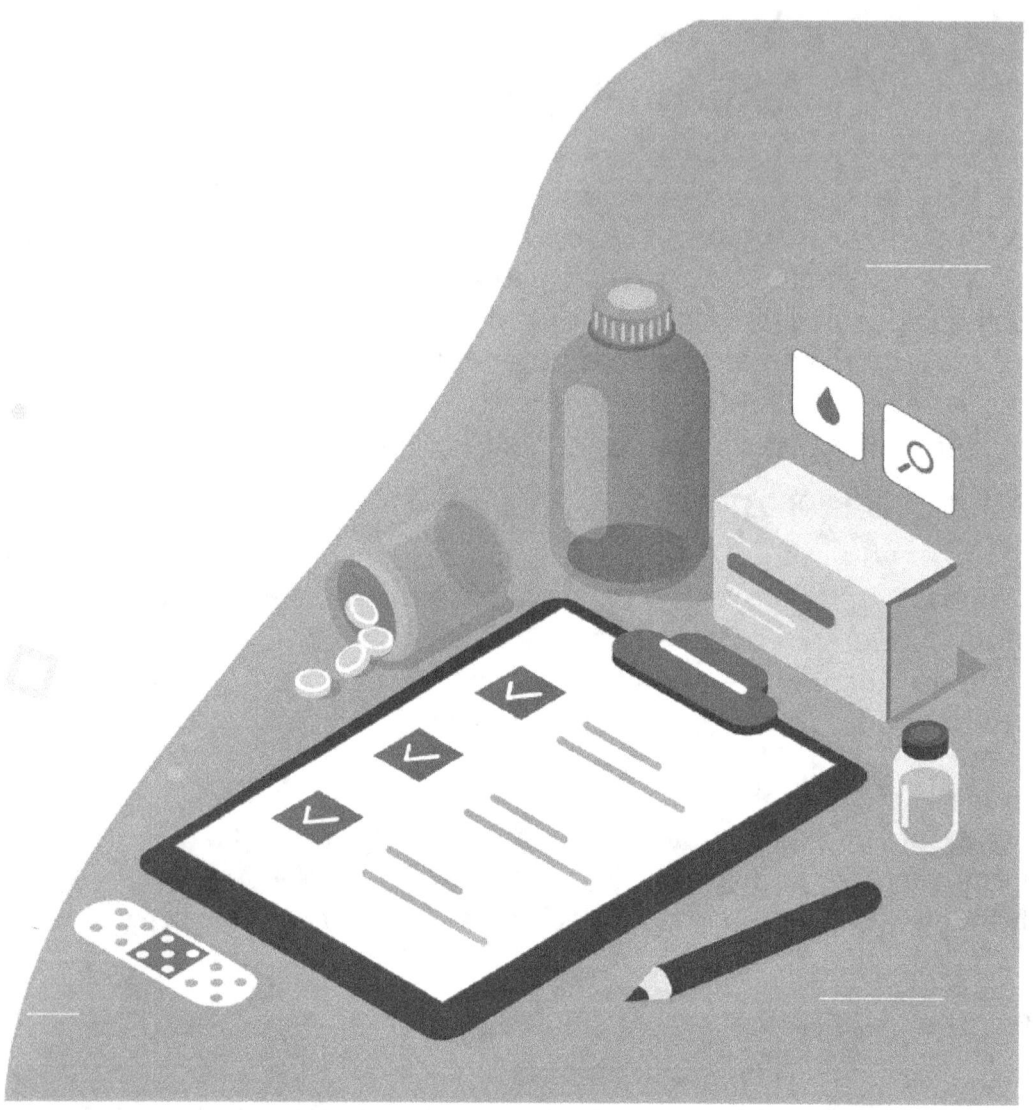

Record dietary habits

Sometimes your LO's food preferences change, and they start eating less healthy foods, or they may completely shun unhealthy food options. Fluctuations in eating patterns could be due to the progression of their disease, current medications, stress levels, and a myriad of other factors. Because what they eat influences their overall well-being, record your LO's eating habits and share any changes with their doctors.

Track exercise routine

Some patient injuries result from unprecedented accidents that may occur while exercising. Document your LO's physical activity to track injuries and physical improvements. Present your LO's exercise routine to their healthcare providers if it contains any information that may improve the appointment's outcome.

Manage mood fluctuations

While mood fluctuations become common in some individuals as Alzheimer's disease worsens, various drug classes also affect one's mood. Keep track of your LO's mood changes and share any changes that may cause you concern. Your LO's doctor can excavate the root of the changes and devise a suitable solution with adequate information.

Record significant incidents

Stay on the lookout for major occurrences such as your LO getting lost for the first time, uncharacteristic behavior compromising other people's peace, or violating your rights. Document all incidents and share the notes with your LO's doctor.

Create a logbook to keep track of other vital details such as:

- the date you sought help, and the response
- follow up actions
- insurance information
- important contact information

Create a medication list

List every health supplement, prescription, and over-the-counter medication your LO takes, including dosages. Your list should be exhaustive, providing a detailed overview of what symptoms and conditions for which your LO takes each of the drugs listed therein. For added comprehension, you can also include the duration for which your LO has been on each medication and any notable changes during the treatment. Pack that list when going for appointments to help your LO's doctor troubleshoot adverse side effects, avoid harmful drug interactions, and prevent overmedication.

Allow your LO to speak for themself

Medical professionals are responsible for delivering unbiased care for your LO despite their busy schedules. Some healthcare providers tend to cruise through notes, directly interact with the primary caregiver, and completely disregard the patient. Doctors or nurses who choose this way of operating do so because it saves them time, and that way, they quickly get straight answers from you. If you come across a healthcare provider who would rather speak to you and wrap the consultation up quickly, politely remind them that your LO is still capable of answering for themself.

Remember that your presence during the scheduled hospital visits is so you can support your LO, not take over their appointment. Your LO might dislike you interfering with their appointment and speak up right then, resulting in hurt feelings or disorder. In other instances, people who do not talk much may just bottle it up internally, slowly fermenting it into resentment before completely shutting down.

Your LO wants to be treated as an adult who can contribute to decisions regarding their own care regardless of how flawed or unreasonable their behavior may sometimes be.

The biggest thing I have learned is to make sure I include my mom in all the conversations related to her condition. I *never* talk to her doctor as if my mom is not in the room. I ask her for permission to share personal details every time. When the doctor asks for a decision, I wait to see if she has an opinion, *then* I offer my view and get her buy-in.

Questions to Ask

While healthcare providers try to give LOs and caregivers most of the essential information regarding conditions, treatment, and follow-up plans, they may inadvertently leave you unfilled gaps. The caregiver asking the right questions for further comprehension goes a long way to understanding. Next are some questions you can ask your LO's doctor to ensure you negate any possibility of confusion.

- What treatments are available?
- Understand every medicine, what it does, how it works, and what kind of side effects it has.
- Prepare a list of any supplements and medications your LO is already taking so the doctor can keep that in mind and prescribe the most suitable treatment.
- What are the side effects?
- Is it long-term?
- Does the dosage change over time?
- What does the disease progression look like?
- Are there stages?
- At which stage will they need regular care, either in-home or in a facility?
- What is a good cadence for follow-up appointments?
- When should we call you?
- What are some non-medical support resources your LO can engage in?
- Is the disease hereditary, and if so, what are suggestions for future generations?

- Will you and your LO work with a dedicated medical professional or a team of doctors and nurses?
- If hospitalization is required, how will the doctor be notified and be able to assist?
- Does the care facility have an online portal that tracks visits, medicines, and after-visit summaries?
- What other complications or illnesses are typical of Alzheimer's diagnosis?

Dissecting Communication Problems

When communicating with doctors, an issue often arises because our LOs won't always tell their doctors the whole truth. This is not meant to criticize or disparage our LOs; instead, if you are currently caregiving, chances are you already have some experience with this phenomenon. Sometimes it's more about showing the truth rather than telling it. LOs may complain about being in pain or show signs that suggest deterioration when only with you, but when they talk to their doctors, they forget or even deny having had any difficulties. Doctors are trained to identify signs and symptoms, but it can spiral into a major caregiving challenge when our LOs hide their symptoms because the doctor can only do so much.

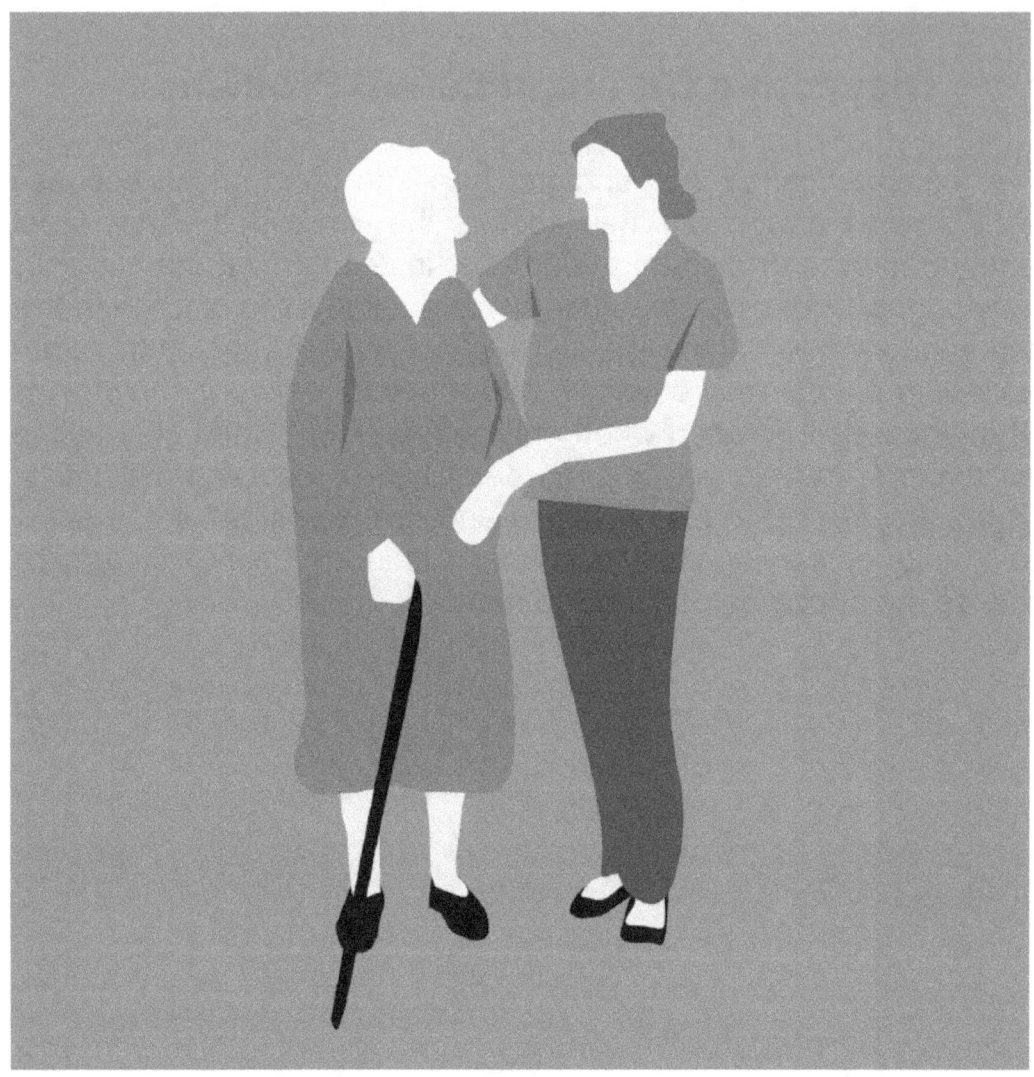

People may mislead their healthcare providers for various reasons ranging from embarrassment to denial, among various other factors. Some of those factors may include:

Fear

The diagnosis of Alzheimer's disease alone is devastating enough, and sometimes elders cover up their actual symptoms for fear of being diagnosed with other related conditions. They feel they have already been through enough and deserve some respite. Our LOs may also downplay their symptoms to avoid what they think is a lousy checkup. In various other cases, LOs feel so bad they are afraid that they may increase the weight of the burden on your shoulders if they face reality.

Embarrassment

LOs may also withhold critical details regarding the progression of their condition to avoid embarrassing or shameful moments. They may think that their doctor might judge them if they were to say everything as it is, so they alter facts to preserve their dignity. Seniors may not want to be seen as weak, deteriorating, or compromised, and a *harmless* lie might seem like a perfect solution.

Denial

We all experience feelings of denial at one point, and so do our LOs. They may sometimes ignore reality and stay in their own perfect dimension where Alzheimer's disease does not exist. It is often observed, especially in the later stages, where they create a slightly alternate reality and, as an example, joyfully tell outsiders stories about their dog when they actually have a cat. This denial strategy often helps them forge past difficult moments throughout the progression of their disease.

The Fault in the Problem

Whether your LO gives their healthcare provider incorrect feedback to feel they are recovering or does so due to fear of embarrassment, misleading information is a step backward. Doctors can only work their miracles when they have enough information to relate to, and when our LOs withhold that information, they make their doctor's job difficult. If healthcare professionals fail to deliver the help needed, your role as a caregiver becomes more problematic because you would have to deal with untreated symptoms that may worsen with time.

You will have to intervene if you find yourself in this problematic situation. Fortunately, you can take some steps to ensure your LO's healthcare team is well-informed without making your LO feel disregarded.

Follow the law

Discuss with family members to secure legal paperwork on time. Get proper authorization and keep a valid power of attorney document in place. Provide copies of essential documents such as power of attorney and advance care directives to the healthcare professionals working on your LO's case.

Discuss communication issues ahead of time

Calm and prepare your LO ahead of time by explaining how today's medical care services differ from options available in the past. Let them know that the healthcare professionals respect patient views and decisions, so close and transparent cooperation with doctors and nurses helps the outcome of their appointment. When your LO understands that asking questions and suggesting opinions is their right as a patient, they may feel more encouraged to open up without fear of being judged.

Build trust as an advocate

Explain your role as your LO's advocate by showing them that you are on their side. Sometimes when people have little faith in their caregivers, they may withdraw details to protect themselves. Remind them that their health and safety are your major priorities, and you want them to receive the best care possible. Once you gain your LO's trust and establish that you are on the same team, encourage them to cooperate without fear, shame, or hesitation.

Send documentation in advance

An efficient trick to quicken the duration of your hospital visit is to send documentation to your LO's doctor before your scheduled visit. Communicate all your concerns when you send the documents. When you arrive at the doctor's office for your LO's scheduled appointment, you will find the doctor ready with the most required facts. Sending documents beforehand quickens the consultation process and decreases the chances of your LO misleading their physician.

Privately warn the doctor beforehand

If you cannot send documentation in advance, ask to speak to the doctor in the absence of your LO and warn them about your LO's tendency to play down symptoms and act "normal." Discuss changes in behavior and any other new symptoms your LO exhibits. While going behind your LO's back may sound uncomfortable, it becomes acceptable in such a case when the patient is limiting the amount of care they receive due to fear, denial, or deteriorating memory. You can talk to their doctor via a call before your hospital visit or discreetly ask to see them in person before they attend to your LO.

Chapter 5:

Navigating Legal and Financial Hurdles

It never occurred to me to put some of this in place years ago; I wouldn't even have known where to start.

—Mom

Sometimes, we ignore essential discussions because we do not want to face reality. We avoid end-of-life discussions with our family and LOs because even the thought of losing them scares and profoundly saddens us. The old adage, "Better to have it and not need it than to need it and not have it," could not be further from the truth when it concerns certain legal and financial matters. Let's accept our current reality, discuss the unimaginable, and get our affairs in order.

The laws that govern legal decisions vary from place to place, and some states require you to go through various channels for some things, which can be overwhelming. To protect your LO's assets and avoid family disputes, involved individuals should dedicate time to explore and make informed legal decisions thoroughly.

Estate Planning

Deciding and creating a plan that states how and by whom one would want their affairs handled when they cannot address the issues on their own is called *Estate Planning*. The plan also makes known who will eventually receive one's assets when nature takes its course.

Estate planning is an overwhelming legal process, but you can dedicate some time to learning and understanding the legal proceedings to encourage your LO to start planning or help them plan.

The first step in estate planning is reviewing estate assets such as:

- land
- investments
- cash
- jewelry
- clothes
- retirement accounts
- cars
- houses
- savings

Estate planning encompasses several components that clearly represent your directive, ensuring your property and other matters are handled as you wish and avoiding misconceptions and disagreements. Let us look into some standard documents to prepare a proper estate plan.

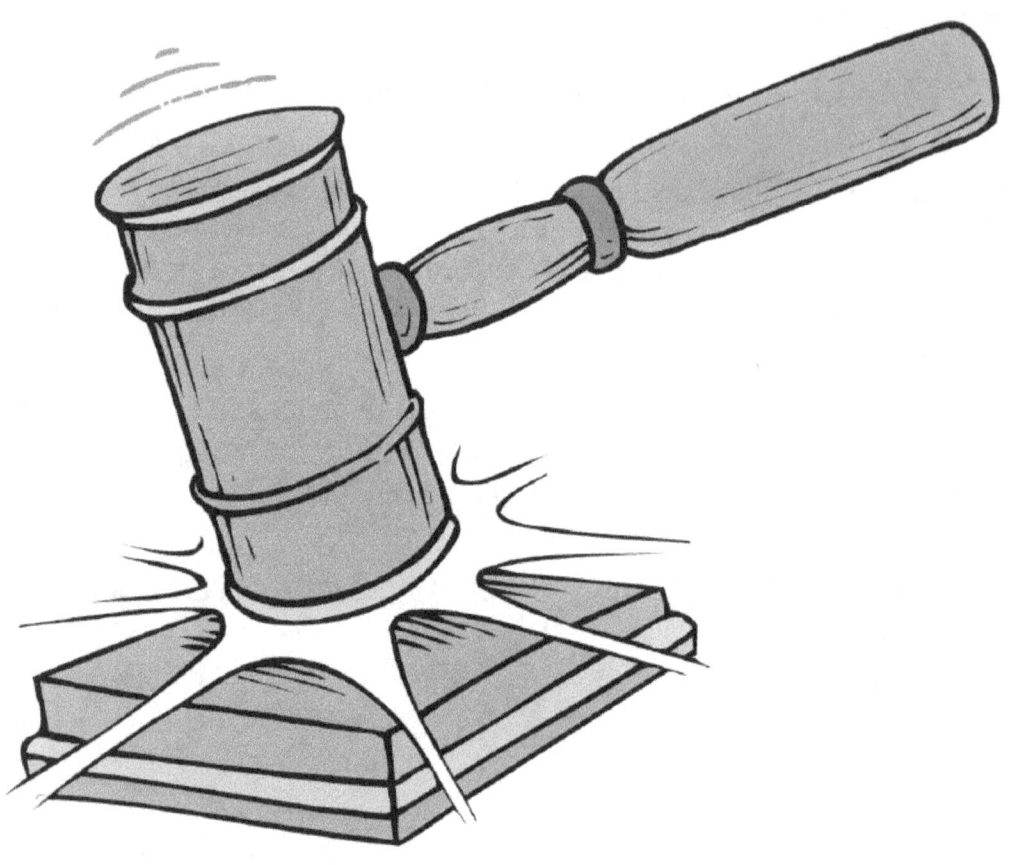

Story Time – "… decisions can be taken away from you."

At some point down my caregiving journey, I needed to arrange oral health care for my mom with a new oral surgeon. We had visited him for the first time as a referral from my regular dentist and did not know what to expect. My mom and I really liked his approach and how comfortable she felt with him as her care provider. She didn't notice, but he figured out quite early in the conversation that my mom had some memory issues. He would direct his questions to my mom and discreetly glance up at me, where I would gently shake or nod my head. During the consultation, he took me aside and asked if I had a healthcare power of attorney. When I told him I hadn't gotten it yet, he declared, "You'd be surprised how quickly those decisions can be taken away from you."

His words struck me like a ton of bricks, and that was the first bit of advice I received that prompted me to spring into action. I learned it was too late for some things as my mom now has a pre-existing condition. Contrary to what I initially thought, it's not enough to have the passwords to your LO's online banking accounts and other business affairs. You need more support; you need the law. I compiled some important things for you regarding legal and financial issues I wish I knew before it was too late.

Power of Attorney

One of the most important legal documents to keep is a *Power of Attorney* document. It gives you the legal capacity to decide and act on behalf of your LO. As its name suggests, it is not just a piece of paper; it is authority. Legal documents that give an individual legal capacity to act and/or decide on behalf of their LO come in different forms, depending on the intended purpose. Your LO can require two different forms and appoint two other individuals, attorneys or agents. In instances where your LO's other caregiver is knowledgeable about the law and finance, that individual can receive legal authority to manage your LO's legal and financial matters while you handle health-related issues. Most power of attorney types may have other names depending on where you live.

Healthcare Power of Attorney

A *Medical Power of Attorney,* also called *Healthcare Power of Attorney* or *Advance Healthcare Directive,* is an essential document that gives you legal authority to make sound decisions about your LO's medical care. It legalizes you to decide treatment options, surgery, end-of-life care, and other healthcare-related issues. Ensure open communication with your LO about healthcare wishes while they can still make sound decisions and get it in writing.

Healthcare power of attorney creates peace of mind for you, your LO, and other individuals involved. Many individuals choose a durable medical power of attorney over a non-durable one. A durable medical power of attorney allows you to retain decision-making authority even after your LO becomes incapacitated in the eyes of the law. Although many courts assume that a medical power of attorney is durable by default, that is not always the case, so your LO should specify when creating the document.

People living with Alzheimer's disease may become too incapacitated to make legal decisions as time goes on. If that happens before they secure critical legal documents, it may cause complications in their care and your peace of mind. In other instances, LOs may still have the mental capacity to create these legal documents but choose not to. Their refusal or inability to sign the legal paperwork leaves you and other involved individuals with few options.

Financial Power of Attorney

A particular type of power of attorney that authorizes you to make financial decisions on behalf of your LO is called a *Financial Power of Attorney*.

Once the power of attorney proceedings are complete, you receive the original document to present to third parties as evidence of your authority to act on behalf of your LO. Depending on its wording, the document can either become effective immediately or upon the occurrence of a specified, future event.

The authority bestowed to you by a valid power of attorney document always ends upon the principal's death; the individual who signs authority over to you. Unless otherwise specified in writing, a power of attorney document becomes invalid if the principal becomes mentally incompetent to make sound legal or financial decisions. The court can invalidate the power of attorney if the principal revokes it or, in divorce cases, the agent was the spouse.

What financial decisions you can make as an agent depends on what your LO authorized in writing. Common powers give you authority to participate in:

- government benefits such as unemployment compensation
- tax issues
- personal property transactions
- claims and litigation
- stock, bond, or other securities transactions
- making gifts to individuals or charities
- estate, trust, and other beneficiary transactions
- handling the operation of a business
- safe deposit box access
- insurance and annuity transactions
- real property transactions
- banking and other financial institution transactions
- retirement benefits

Power of Attorney Challenges

In the most fortunate scenario, your LO planned ahead and secured the necessary legal documents before their doctor could label them as mentally incompetent. However, it is not that simple under other circumstances. Find out how to navigate some common scenarios that may impact the legal part of your caregiving journey.

Scenario 1: It's too late for your LO to sign a power of attorney document.

Diminished mental capacity is a matter of when not if. When your LO loses the ability to remember important details such as who their family is or who they would want to make decisions on their behalf, they no longer have the competence to sign the power of attorney documents.

There is little you can do other than apply for formal guardianship if this is your case. Also called conservatorship, formal guardianship is the power the court gives you to manage your LO's care and maintenance. However, the legal procedures you would have to carry out to get this kind of guardianship are expensive and time-consuming due to court costs, agents' fees, and legal fees.

Option: Use your marital status to maintain access to co-owned assets.

If you are legally married to your LO and you, as a couple, have decided to hold your assets as co-owners, then you can still access assets and financial accounts without going through the guardianship hustle.

Scenario 2: The person is mentally able but refuses to sign a power of attorney document.

In this scenario, your LO is still entitled to make personal healthcare and financial decisions, and if they refuse to sign the power of attorney documents, there is very little you can do to help them.

If the problem is trust, encourage them to designate someone they can trust for the decision-making role. In some instances, they may choose to entirely ignore estate planning decisions, which creates a challenging situation for involved parties.

First Option: Suggest standby guardianship instead.

Have an honest discussion about the importance of having healthcare or financial power of attorney, explore the disadvantages of ignoring such necessary documentation, and give your LO time to take your advice, weigh the consequences, and decide.

Your LO listens to reason and agrees to proceed with the legal planning, or they maintain their perspective. If giving power of attorney remains a challenging idea, suggest standby guardianship instead. It is typically less burdensome to have your LO agree to sign the documents willingly than involuntary guardianship. Explain how standby guardianship works and allow them time to mull it over.

If your LO still refuses to act, your last option is to apply to the court for involuntary guardianship so you can help them make better decisions.

Second Option: Emphasize that the process is not about age.

Explain to your LO that these documents should be secured as a preparedness measure, not necessarily because they are older. We are talking about early-onset Alzheimer's disease, after all. Use examples if you can think of any. Your LO might feel more relaxed knowing that other people have taken steps to put these documents in place regardless of age.

Guardianship

If your LO is no longer capable of caring for themself, and the rest of their family disagrees on the type of care required, or there is no family, the court can, at your request, appoint a guardian to make decisions for your LO.

Obtaining a *Guardianship* entails hiring counsel and testifying in court during guardianship hearings and is not a one-day process, so you would have to prepare yourself for multiple trips to and from government offices.

Not only does guardianship entitle you to handle healthcare and financial decisions for your LO, but the court will hold you accountable for your LO's fundamental requirements for safety, care, food, and shelter.

The laws and processes for guardianship-related matters differ from state to state, so if you would like to apply for guardianship, you can speak to an elder care attorney experienced with the guardianship process in your state. Have your LO declare what they want to happen and who they want to look after any of their dependents if they can no longer do so themself. Guardianship instructions are usually included in a part of their *will*, another estate planning document explained next.

Will

Unlike a *Living Will*, a *Will* is a legal document that defines your LO's appointed executor and beneficiaries in the event of their death. This document is mainly about your LO's final wishes regarding estate administration and does not communicate healthcare choices. It is wise to put a signed will in place as soon as possible, regardless of how the disease progresses. Preparedness has little to do about

Alzheimer's disease itself, but your peace of mind and your LO's comfort in knowing they have communicated their final wishes.

When dealing with wills, you will often encounter words such as *executor* and *beneficiary*. An executor is a person in charge of the estate's administration, while beneficiaries are the individuals who will receive the estate's assets. The appointed executor specified in the will only gain legal authority over the estate in the event of your LO's death.

Again, the legality of a will differs from state to state, so you might want to check your local regulations to help your LO set up their will.

Living Trust

Another way for your LO to communicate instructions on managing or disposing of their estate after their death is through a *Living Trust*. Depending on state laws and other court-related factors, a living trust may allow an estate to avoid probate, a quality that makes a living trust more convenient than wills.

Once your LO sets up a living trust, they transfer ownership of the included property but retain control while they live. The living trust can consist of valuable assets such as their stocks, home, jewels, and bank accounts. Your LO can also designate a custodian to manage the assets they leave for minor children through a living trust.

Your LO names a *trustee*, one who will be in charge of holding the trust's assets and administering them according to the instructions from your LO and for the benefit of the trust's beneficiaries. They can name themself as the initial trustee since they do not have much cognitive damage at this point in the progression of the disease. That means they retain complete control over the property and can use it as they see fit. In the event of their death, a *successor trustee*, appointed by your LO when setting up the trust, takes over and shares the trust property with your LO's beneficiaries as directed. Living trusts can be categorized into two main types, as briefly covered next.

Revocable Living Trust

The most common and flexible form of living trust available, the *Revocable Living Trust*, is often what most people mean when talking about trusts in general. Your LO can amend or cancel the trust if they find it necessary. They can also add more property to the trust, sell the assets mentioned therein, or amend the guidelines. A revocable living trust eliminates the trouble of dealing with an unreliable successor trustee in the future because your LO can make amendments and choose someone different, should they and their team notice concerning behavior changes.

Irrevocable Living Trust

With *Irrevocable Trusts*, your LO cannot amend guidelines, sell trust property, or alter the beneficiaries as they wish. Should the need to amend the trust become inevitable, your LO would need all the beneficiaries to agree to changes on paper or discuss the matter with a judge.

Irrevocable trusts are a little more complex and less prevalent than revocable ones. They can also help to benefit from estate tax-saving strategies if one transfers assets from their taxable estate to an irrevocable trust. Irrevocable trusts are more advantageous to individuals whose estates exceed the federal estate tax exemption.

Life Insurance

Life insurance is yet another essential thing your LO must secure while they still have time, so it's good to buy it as soon as possible. If they didn't already have one in place and have an Alzheimer's diagnosis, they are no longer eligible for standard life insurance, but there are other options to consider.

Guaranteed Issue Insurance

This form of life insurance does not request any health information or require a medical examination from applicants. It may, however, come with a graded period, a time when the total coverage amount is not available at the beginning of their policy. The graded period is usually the first two or three years from obtaining the insurance. If they pass away during this graded period, their beneficiaries only receive a return of the premiums paid, not the policy's face value.

Simplified Issue Insurance

This sort of life insurance asks only a few questions about your LO's health before getting them on board. This plan is ideal for individuals who do not want to undergo a medical examination or those who need immediate coverage.

Simplified Issue Life insurance provides a small coverage amount much faster than traditional policies. The difference in lead time is primarily because with simplified issue insurance, there is no need for a comprehensive medical examination. The majority of individuals who apply for this type of insurance usually gain coverage within a few days, that is, once the company approves the application for the insurance policy.

From the few questions they ask, companies that offer simplified issue insurance will be able to assess risk and determine a premium and death benefit. Your LO may be able to choose between permanent coverage and term policy, depending on which company they choose.

Remember that the simplified life insurance policy would be the best fit if:

- One needs life insurance but does not want to undergo a medical exam.
- One needs coverage as soon as possible, without having to wait.
- One has been ordered by the court to get life insurance right away.
- One needs collateral for a loan, and a life insurance policy may serve as collateral.
- One's term policy has run out, and they need to keep it as they figure out what to do next.
- One requires life insurance but is unsure if one would qualify for standard policies.

Remember that it is better to have life insurance in place and not need it than need it and not have it.

The Cost of Not Planning

Advance planning offers multiple advantages, such as your LO making informed decisions after thoroughly contemplating who would make the best decisions on their behalf, with their interests in mind and at heart. Discussing power of attorney proceedings in advance also lets your LO decide when the authorities should become effective. Another benefit of prior planning is that involved parties can revise the documents whenever necessary, as long as your LO is mentally competent.

What happens if the need arises to use the legal documents, but they are not in place? Discord. Apart from family members disagreeing on specific treatment options or financial decisions, lack of legal preparedness puts your LO and other concerned parties at the risk of deception. Several family members report abuse involving their LO being deprived of basic care by their agent or assets being liquidated for the agent's personal gain. Although difficult to imagine, some children extort their parents without shame. Some spouses emotionally divorce their partners when faced with hardships but stay in the communion to milk as many financial benefits as possible.

Usually, an individual knows their family and friends well. They know who to trust and who not to, but involved parties often make legal decisions in haste when there was no prior legal planning.

The cost of NOT planning could leave your LO with nothing to their name or their beneficiaries with nothing to inherit or leave those remaining with mountains of legal troubles and debt to sort out the estate. With that, I urge you to act as soon as possible, and then you and your LO can check it off the list!

Chapter 6:

Finding Your Peace

At this point, we've discussed what Alzheimer's disease and caregiving are and what responsibilities you may gain, including the best way to stay ahead of the myriad of medical, legal, and financial decisions you may have to help make. This chapter intends to encourage you to find what puts YOU at peace to be the best caregiver for your LO and avoid burning yourself out. I know you could relate if someone shared their story and told you they cannot remember the last time they went out with friends or did anything that felt good in any other situation. Similarly, it is heartbreaking to see a fellow caregiver break into tears, weak to their knees, and lament that caregiving took over life, and now they just live to take care of their LO.

Most of us experience this profound hopelessness more often than we care to admit. We must learn to comfort ourselves because we are all our LOs have in some cases. We shove our pain and resentment down deep and carry on, completely ignoring the harm it causes us. But what if it does not have to be that way? What do we do when caregiving hurts so badly it takes over our mental health and drives our general well-being off the cliff? Would you believe me if I told you there is another way? This chapter will cover caregiving stress and depression and explore ways to find peace, perform self-care, and "put on your oxygen mask before helping others."

Stress and Depression

Stress and depression are easily every Alzheimer's caregiver's nightmare. I put together some of the common signs accompanying stress or depression in caregiving.

Denial

It is pervasive for caregivers to spiral into denial about the disease and how much it changes the reality of life with their LO. Caregivers in denial often comfort themselves that it's just a passing phase and their LO will get better soon. Denial hits other caregivers initially when their LO's doctor passes the diagnosis or when their LO shares it. They would convince themselves that the healthcare provider is mistaken, that it simply cannot be. Have you ever felt that way?

Denial presents itself differently in different individuals because we process emotions uniquely. If you are experiencing signs of denial, you can soar above it by accepting the reality. Although cruel and brutal to accept, this is the new normal, and avoiding the truth only hinders your caregiving journey, robbing you of the special time you could spend with your LO.

Anger

Taking care of someone with cognitive difficulties can be highly challenging and triggers a range of emotions in caregivers, including anger. We are only human, and getting upset, angry, frustrated, resentful, or even having feelings of guilt is a normal reaction. But does it help your LO? Not at all. Whether you get mad and snap, or you get angry and bottle it up, the fact remains that your LO needs help to carry out tasks that a healthy individual their age would be able to accomplish without help.

Yes, It is tiresome and frustrating, but you are who they have. You are their anchor, and they look to you for help whenever they encounter an obstacle. Even if your LO does not ask for help, but you realize they need assistance, offer to help them.

No one wants to be a burden or be perceived as one, including your LO. If they say they need help to make up the bed because they can't tell which side of the sheet is the inside, that is no laughing matter, and they are not proud to come up to you seeking help for such a simple task. Fortunately, many individuals in the early stages of the disease still have most of their abilities, so they may need help with only a few errands.

Try not to show irritation or anger. Our faces usually betray us in situations like these. Although your LO may not say anything about it, they notice, and you don't want them to feel the difference in your attitude toward them.

Social Withdrawal

If only we could add more hours to our 24 hour-days! With the highly demanding duties you have as a caregiver, time to engage with friends or participate in self-care activities outside your caregiving perimeter can become an unaffordable luxury. You may withdraw from hanging out with your friends, neighbors, or colleagues due to a tight schedule.

Apart from time, caregivers withdraw from social activities because they feel as though they no longer belong with people who were previously in their circle of friends. The feeling of displacement is either due to caregivers thinking that no one would understand what they are going through or fear that no one would still want to interact with them. Do you often avoid social interaction because you think you do not fit in with your friends and neighbors anymore?

Although there is not much we can do about time apart from proper scheduling and canceling less important activities to make time for essential ones, we can definitely fight the feeling of displacement.

You are a wonderful person. Draw a breath, close your eyes, and breathe out. Let that sink into your mind and body. Breathe out and open your eyes. Stepping up to take care of your LO at their most needful time makes you a good person, and going the extra mile to learn more about how to take care of them from *This Book* makes you an exceptional caregiver. Remember that and distance yourself from anyone who thinks caregiving nibbles at your value because it does the opposite. You are enough; don't let anyone or anything convince you otherwise.

Anxiety

What if I am not there someday? What if I can no longer provide for them? What if..

You prove me right in saying that you are an excellent caregiver if you tend to get lost in thoughts, wondering about the future. Many caregivers spend time envisioning their LO's future without help but confess that the images are bleak and inconclusive.

Anxiety only sways you toward caregiver depression. Although it is a normal part of caregiving to worry, constant, uncontrollable anxiety is harmful to your health. If conflicted questions and worries about the future overtake your mind and body, taking up most of your caregiving and self-care time, recognize you are spiraling, take a moment, and redirect the feelings into something more productive.

Exhaustion

Exhaustion interferes with your caregiving duties because if your LO needs assistance, but you have not addressed your need for rest, then your LO cannot always rely on you for support.

Many caregivers admit having turned down their LO more than once because they were too tired to help. Your roles as a caregiver only increase with time, and I wish I could tell you it gets less tiresome, but that would be insincere, and we are here to talk about your new realities. You can, however, look into ways of organizing your schedule and try grouping tasks according to priority.

Sleeplessness

Constant anxiety can lead to sleepless nights. You may spend too much time wondering what might happen to your LO at night or how their mood will be the next day. It becomes difficult to fall asleep when one has so much conflict within themself. But what happens when you deprive yourself of needed sleep? What are the consequences of irregular sleep patterns? What about the effects of insufficient sleep on your health?

If you tend to lose sleep over thoughts, work, or constant fear, you might want to reevaluate your priorities and reorganize your sleep schedule. Lack of sleep causes confusion, dizziness, fatigue, headaches, and many other symptoms you do not want to encounter when your LO needs you by their side.

Some caregivers admit having had to cut a few hours off of their sleep schedule to accommodate the needs of their LO. The sacrifice is as heartwarming as it is heart-wrenching because it puts you at risk for many problems that will not stop at caregiving stress and depression but also compromise your capacity as a caregiver.

Irritability

Have you ever snapped at your LO out of frustration? I admit I am completely guilty of having a short fuse. Maybe you've never clipped your responses to your LO, but what about harshly responding to other people because you had too much on your mind? It's cruel what caregiving stress can do to us.

While it is normal and acceptable to drown in your thoughts once in a while, unjustifiable negative responses and actions could cross the line. If you are easily triggered, have trouble controlling your mood, or often feel as though everyone is out to annoy you, you will likely simply need more sleep.

Many caregivers become irritable because the job is demanding; they have no time to breathe and sometimes, no one to share the burden with. That kind of pressure is so powerful it can change one into something unrecognizable when they look at their reflection in the mirror.

Lack of Concentration

Sometimes caregivers get so busy taking care of their LOs that they forget to attend to other equally important tasks. The stress of caregiving can attack you from the core, then slowly work toward the outside, making you less and less efficient. If you become forgetful because there is a lot to do, how much confidence do you have to care for your LO who forgets things? How would it reflect on your caregiving skills if your LO got hurt because you got busy with laundry and forgot to dry the floor after spilling water? I know it sounds terrible, but it happens, and we have to talk about it, so it cannot happen to you.

Stressed caregivers lose concentration, and it can affect all aspects of life; home, work, school, etc., but the most important part is recognizing it. Many become so lost they do not even realize their caregiving skills are becoming sub-par. If you often lose concentration and neglect matters that need your attention because you get busy with other tasks, you may need to improve your concentration.

Depression

This is a mega concern; caregiving depression is sour, cruel, and fatal. Several caregivers exhibit signs of depression and don't even realize it. It affects each individual differently. More severe than dietary changes and darker than constant feelings of guilt, depressed caregivers are at risk of engaging in self-harm. Caregiving depression is real, and if you are experiencing symptoms, know that there is no shame in admitting it, you are not alone, and help is available. If you feel you have given too much into caregiving and have nothing left to sacrifice, know that the condition is treatable. Many caregivers recover and get back on their feet even stronger than before, and if you find the strength to read This Book remember to remind yourself that YOU matter.

Seeing the Doctor

Please see your physician if you regularly experience signs of caregiving stress or believe you might be depressed. Untreated depression interferes with the quality of care you can deliver to your LO, so do not postpone your visit to the doctor on account of caregiving. This is an emergency! Before you panic, some medical conditions and medications can cause symptoms of depression and stress. It does not necessarily mean the source is caregiving pressure if you are stressed, but that also does not make the matter any lighter. You still need a doctor to rule out possibilities and suggest a way forward.

Once your healthcare provider confirms depression, treatment is the next step. Depending on the cause, treatment for depression often revolves around therapy, support, and medication. The earlier you start treatment, the faster you can feel better and resume positive caregiving.

If your doctor prescribed medication, bear in mind that your body will process it differently, affecting your recovery period. Depending on how well your body reacts to the medication, it can take up to a month before you completely recover. Remember to discuss side effects with your healthcare provider to avoid surprises when you get home and start feeling like the medication worsens your situation.

Counseling

For counseling, your doctor may recommend that you work with a psychologist, social worker, psychiatrist, counselor, or any mental health expert who would deliver the most appropriate treatment plan, depending on how much help you need. One major thing to remember is that whichever mental health professional you end up with should be one you can openly communicate with. Some experts naturally look judgmental even before they part their lips to speak. Sometimes it's just in our heads, but other times they really do look through us and silently weigh our every decision.

The Extra Mile

Professional assistance is not the only way out of depression. You can make efforts to cope with your situation as a caregiver, such as accepting help from family and friends, seeking caregiver support, and participating in activities you enjoy. You can also attempt recording your feelings in a diary or notebook. The exercise of recording both positive and negative emotions can work like talk therapy; it gives you an outlet where judgment is nonexistent because it is just you and your journal. Give yourself time to relax and engage in self-care activities that help reduce stress.

Control your stress level

Stress can cause blurred vision, elevated blood pressure, and appetite fluctuations, among other effects. All these can hinder your caregiving progress, so you may want to control your stress levels. You can engage in relaxing activities to calm your mind and set your thoughts straight. Remember to consult your doctor if you notice any concerning symptoms.

Be practical

You being there for your LO makes a difference. A huge difference. However, you may lose control of your body and mind if you do not realize that many behaviors are beyond your control. Not everything that goes wrong down this path is your fault. In that same manner, you cannot control everything that happens because some things are beyond us. Let go of the negative things that happen to you or your LO, make peace with your LO's misgivings, and focus on the positive moments, savoring each gain with delight.

Recognize your effort

Appreciate your effort. Keep in mind that you play a significant role in the life of your LO. You don't have to be perfect. No one does everything right all of the time, and accepting that can save you an ounce of heartbreak. Do not punish yourself by wondering what you could have done better because sometimes we do everything right and still hit obstacles hard before tumbling down.

Allow yourself to relax

Take personal time off from your daily caregiving duties. Allow yourself to be selfish for a few hours and take that time to relax. It's natural to feel you need a break from your caring responsibilities.

Listen to your body and take that break if you feel that way. Some do not even realize they need a break until it's too late, and caregiver burnout has taken its toll on their health.

<u>Accept change as it comes</u>

There is no way to predict the exact changes that await your LO and the time they will manifest. Prepare to accept change as it comes. That way, you reduce pressure on yourself because you worry less about what tomorrow holds for your LO and equip yourself to face new changes and adjust as your situation requires.

The Change

Whether the person battling Alzheimer's disease is your parent, friend, or spouse, you will experience a dynamic shift of responsibilities in your relationship. How many friends help their friends pick clothes daily when there is no special event to attend? Honestly, the change is sudden and can be confusing, but how do we make peace with it? How do we carry on knowing our responsibilities increase with the progression of the disease? We prepare. We adjust. We maximize every moment.

Work and Business

While some caregivers prepare for significant changes to their work schedules or change jobs completely, others prepare to take on new jobs in addition to their current positions. Change is change, regardless of the direction. When work pressure meets caregiving stress, one may be forced to make a difficult choice between their job or taking care of their LO. In other cases, caregivers work two jobs to make ends meet. If you have to pay for your LO's medical bills and other living expenses but know that the math does not agree with your bank balance, piling jobs on yourself might not be the solution because too much pressure contributes to caregiving stress.

Plan your budget considering all the expenses for which you are responsible. Once you know how much you and your LO need and how far it takes you, compare it against your income or the period in question and decide from there. Still not balancing. Prepare to improvise. Find any expenses you can cut or items you can do without. If you and your LO are living in different areas, analyze how much money it would save you if one of you were to move closer to the other or, if both of you would be comfortable, move in together.

Intimacy

If the individual suffering from Alzheimer's disease is your spouse, you can be distraught at the changes in your intimate relationship. You may feel the physical or emotional connection you once had fading away, watch your LO grow distant, and you may question your role in their life. These emotions and questions are expected and do not make you selfish.

Prepare for changes in your LO's libido because individuals battling Alzheimer's disease often experience changes in sexual desire. The decrease in sexual interest is usually due to some of their medication, depression, and physical sickness. The dramatic shift from being an intimate partner to being a caregiver can sometimes be overwhelming. However, the good thing is that there are still other ways through which you can connect with your LO and make your relationship live again.

Family and Friends

Prepare for your social circle to shrink inward. Your family and friends may be hesitant to spend time with you and your LO because they are unsure how to interact or help. You would be surprised how many people do not know how to comfort their friends in times of need. Some people have no idea how to express their feelings, which does not make them unconcerned. Other people may also feel that they can only help by giving you space, so they draw lines and watch you from afar. It may sound strange but try to remember that we all have different ways of processing things, so your friends and family growing distant could be their way of showing you they care, not the opposite.

Some people may find your LO's changes in behavior a little unsettling and may not know how to communicate with them. Help them understand how your LO's mind now works and provide them with practical communication tips. For family members who want to help but do not know how, provide them with ways in which they can help, suggest tasks, and invite them to spend more time with you and your LO.

What about those who intentionally distance themselves? Accept that not everyone is as strong as you are. Many people out in the world wouldn't last a day in your shoes. Try to see the situation from their perspective and make peace with their decision, because in the end, you need friends who can stand by through any challenge.

Other people, however, have both ignorance and arrogance simmering in their minds, leading me to yet another problematic discussion: How do you handle stigma?

Stigmatization

Do you remember back in the seventies and eighties when people knew so little about the human immunodeficiency virus (HIV) that they would avoid contact with people whose family members had it?

Remember how those diagnosed with HIV would face discrimination from strangers and friends alike due to a lack of knowledge and information? While you may not have had it that bad, other caregivers face intense undeserved judgment in every direction they face, so we cannot sugarcoat this problem. How do you find peace when surrounded by people who can be so close-minded?

Several caregivers and their LOs often worry about being stigmatized. Your LO may feel misunderstood due to other people's misconceptions about the disease. A judgmental environment negatively impacts your role as a caregiver because it can prevent your LO from seeking medical attention when they notice symptoms. They watch in fear as their thinking deteriorates, hoping it all goes away someday.

Stigmatization prevents people from enjoying their lives and making the best of their moments. How can one enjoy spending time out if they cannot even take a sip without people looking at them funny? The same disapproval stops people from participating in clinical trials, which means fewer discoveries and an increased lack of knowledge. Have you or your LO been treated differently because of Alzheimer's disease? How did you respond?

Expressing the Depth

For many caregivers and their LOs, stigma and misconceptions are a substantial barrier to improving their quality of life. The diagnosis of Alzheimer's disease may test friendships and leave affected individuals isolated.

If friends look at you differently because you take care of your LO, you may feel abandoned or blame yourself for their flawed view. Family members may turn on you and avoid discussing the sickness or engaging with you.

Stigma at Work

One would think in today's modern workplace, professionals know better than to discriminate against others based on circumstances beyond human control, but there may be unconscious biases. People with Alzheimer's may lose their jobs because some companies suddenly notice signs of incompetence.

If your or your LO's work environment doesn't support an inclusive culture, you may be at risk of being undermined or disrespected because of their diagnosis. Although your LO only has a few thinking challenges in the early stage of the disease, others may turn your LO down, preferring to work with their colleague instead.

Coping

Here are a few tips to overcome the stigma around Alzheimer's disease.

Be true

Participate in conversations with people about Alzheimer's disease and the need for prevention, better treatment, and a cure. Interact with others who share your interests. Open up and speak your mind, making constructive suggestions as you see fit. Share your experience as a caregiver and discuss the problems you and your LO face due to people's lack of knowledge about Alzheimer's disease.

Share facts

We have established that stigma often results from a lack of knowledge, so you can help educate others by sharing facts and dispelling myths. To do that, you need to have sound knowledge yourself because some individuals may ask difficult questions. Welcome questions with an open mind and understand that the people asking only seek to understand, not judge. Invest some of your free time learning new facts about Alzheimer's disease so you can provide updated information. Participate in the solution by pushing for awareness, more support, and research on Alzheimer's disease.

Believe in yourself

Do not let other people's refusal discourage you. Their reasons and views are not a reflection of you. Stand your ground and let them be if they are unwilling to learn or change their perspective. Remain in touch with those who choose to stay. Hold on to meaningful relationships and strive to make new friends who can relate to what you are going through. Find a support group you can join and maintain the network, sharing experiences with other people in similar situations.

Spread awareness, and fight stigmatization.

What to Remember

Consider treating yourself to some alone time, refresh, and refocus. You can also join Facebook groups to interact with people in similar situations, get realistic advice, and share your experience. Communicating with other people who understand what you are going through helps you find your peace because you realize you are not alone. Remember to count on your healthcare providers and keep up with your own health by honestly sharing concerns with the professionals. Your well-being is a priority too. Talk to someone. At first, you may refrain from sharing your challenges to avoid being perceived as "oversharing," but try talking to someone once you learn which people you can trust. You can talk to your doctor, friend, a member of your team, or a mental health coach. They are there for you, always.

Chapter 7:

Is There Hope?

I'm sorry if you told me already, but why do I have to take THIS pill?
—Mom

Alzheimer's disease is a difficult diagnosis. As a caregiver, it's normal to wonder what exactly is next for your LO. Several caregivers testify they would pay to have their LO's memory restored to experience together everything they missed out on while they were busy with work, school, or business. The primary question stands: Is there hope? The answer depends on how you interpret the information you will learn in this chapter so let us get to it. Please note that the treatments described in this section are current as of the writing of this book. I would encourage you to discuss these options with your LO's healthcare provider to get the most current and relevant information.

Available Treatments

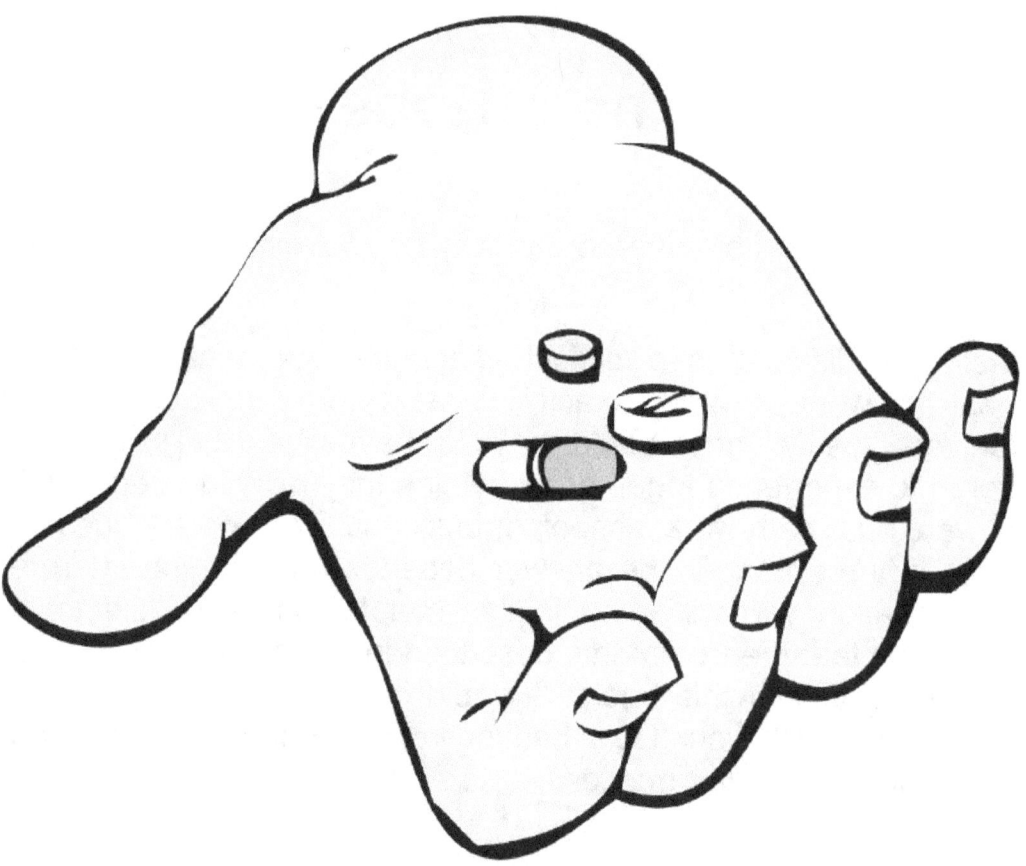

As scientists dive deeper into human body systems and solve biochemistry puzzles, the Food and Drug Administration (FDA) patiently waits to safeguard us from the distribution of unsuitable medications. Some of the FDA-approved drugs used in the early stages of Alzheimer's disease include donepezil (Aricept), rivastigmine (Exelon), and galantamine (Razadyne). With effects lasting six to twelve months, the drugs repress the breakdown of acetylcholine, a brain chemical that facilitates memory and learning.

The FDA also approved aducanumab (Aduhelm) to help reduce amyloid deposits in the brain, resultantly helping slow the progression of Alzheimer's disease (Cummings et al., 2021). Available treatments are not cures; they only ease symptoms in some people by slowing the disease and improving brain functionality. Different drugs work differently in each individual, so it is narrowed down to what works for each patient. The work requires you and your LO to be patient and understanding during the trial period until your healthcare providers establish the best course of treatment. Encourage your LO to be open to their doctor about the symptoms they experience because that helps the physician determine the best treatment option. Some of the factors your LO's doctor considers include the severity of the disease and the patient's age, lifestyle, and preference.

Other Treatments

As Alzheimer's disease advances, your LO might require other medicines to control other symptoms related to the disease, such as insomnia and mood fluctuations. They may also need to alleviate symptoms of other illnesses and often need pain relief medications. The rate at which the body metabolizes and excretes drugs declines with age, which becomes a challenge when aging individuals need to use multiple drugs. This may cause drugs to reach toxic levels in your LO's body, so the chances of a drug overdose are high.

Your LO's physician may hesitate to use drugs that manage behavioral challenges if the risk of complications outweighs the desirable benefits of taking the drugs. To avoid complications, you may want to inform your LO's healthcare provider of everything the patient takes, from herbs to prescription drugs. With time, should your LO need to take other medications for pain or any other symptoms that may accompany the disease, their doctor will refer to the medicines you provided before prescribing anything. Healthcare providers also need to know if their patient takes alcohol, as drinking can also cause complications when it mixes with medications.

One way around common drug complications is by using alternative therapies to combat undesirable symptoms. For example, you can speak to a specialized behavioral therapist about suitable treatments for your LO instead of taking drugs that keep behavioral systems in check.

Sleep Medications

One of the most common issues caregivers experience is that their LOs tend to mix day and evening. People with Alzheimer's disease may become overly active at night, disturbing others who would be trying to rest. Sleep problems can be a significant challenge when they keep occurring because that means you and any other people in the house have to cope with irregular sleep patterns and the headaches and stress that come with it. Many caregivers testify that sleep problems contribute to sending their LOs to nursing facilities, so sleep deprivation is a huge problem.

Sleep medications may cause your LO to feel sleepy during the day. Some drugs may also cause falls and mood changes. Because of the risks associated with prescription or over-the-counter sleeping drugs in people with Alzheimer's, your LO's doctor may be against the self-administration of sleeping tablets. Instead, the doctor may recommend active sleep pattern improvement through bedtime schedules and nighttime activities that improve your LO's sleep quality. We will discuss more bedtime activities in the next chapter so you can discover a range of relaxation ideas to help your LO sleep better at night and maintain regular sleep patterns.

Should there be the need for sedation and no other option exists, try to interact as closely as you can with your LO's healthcare providers. You will need someone with extensive experience and training in the field to help you understand what sleep medication means for your LO. Remember, you are not in this alone, so avoid hopping into a drugstore to buy sleeping tablets before thoroughly discussing it with your LO's doctor.

Antipsychotics and Antidepressants

If your LO exhibits disturbing aggression and extreme anxiety symptoms, antidepressants and antipsychotic medicine can help keep those problems under a leash. Both drugs have common side effects such as constipation, nasal congestion, dry mouth, and incontinence. Adverse side effects vary in different people, and some of the factors that determine how one reacts to specific medication include weight, age, and physical fitness.

Sometimes behavioral problems stem from communication issues at home, problems between you, family members, friends, and the diagnosed. Your LO's healthcare provider will help work through provided information to arrive at the root of issues and devise solutions. In most cases, there will be no need to overwhelm your LO with loads of medication because you just have to improve the level of interaction at home and ensure there is nothing silently troubling your LO.

Behavior medications can take around three to four weeks to reach therapeutic levels in the body, so the results won't be instant. Your LO could worry or panic when they do not notice any improvement but try to calm them down and encourage them to keep taking the drugs as advised until there is a noticeable improvement. Should you see any signs of worsening behavior, immediately alert your LO's doctor.

Other Medications

People who have Alzheimer's disease may also be receiving treatment for other health conditions such as hypertension, heart disease, or diabetes. If that is the case with your LO, be sure to inform their doctor about it so they can keep that in mind.

Vultures Amidst the Pain

Con artists and instant remedy merchants seem to appear out of nowhere when the issue is an incurable illness. They capitalize on people's hopes and concerns, making empty promises about an immediate cure. However, when you look at it from a clear lens, they only seek to make a living out of your pain and false hope. Moreover, most of these bogus "remedies" result in lifelong health complications. Instant remedy salespeople keep their eyes and ears out for their target market—compassionate friends and family desperate to cure incurable conditions and have their LOs back.

When conventional medicine fails to provide hope, concerned individuals may wander searching for other options. Although the internet has been an enormous privilege to this generation, it sometimes presents itself as a curse when it opens doors for deception and misinformation, providing an easy way to lure caregivers with enticing promises. What follows are two of the common features that always accompany false treatments.

Exaggerated language

Watch for dramatic phrasing such as "miracle cure" and "groundbreaking discovery." Producers who are brave and desperate enough even go an extra mile to offer you *a secret remedy that doctors don't want you to know*. Seriously? Why would doctors not want you to know if there was any cure? Are they not toiling with research every day to try and come up with something tangible? If anything, your LO's doctor would keep you from trying false therapies to stop wasting your money and time on something that may even do your LO more harm than good.

Outlandish claims

Manufacturers who claim their product completely cures the devastating effects of unrelated conditions such as Alzheimer's disease, alopecia, arthritis, psoriasis, and diabetes, may have nefarious intentions. Even in this era of technological advancements, there is no such thing as *a cure-all* in the context of Alzheimer's disease.

Clinical Trials

Behind every medical breakthrough that comes to life are groups of skilled people who dedicated their time and energy to sow hope. Clinical trials are a sequence of procedures used to evaluate new strategies to solve medical puzzles to detect, prevent, treat or cure diseases.

Without testing on a subset of the afflicted population, we would have no prevention measures, therapies, or cures for any significant health plagues that once afflicted humanity. It is the same hope we have for a cure for Alzheimer's disease; to stand together and face this disease head-on. To trust the specialists who have dedicated their lives to researching this disease. To believe that their efforts pay off one day, and we go home knowing our LO's participation in clinical trials made it possible.

Unfortunately, finding people willing to participate in clinical trials is a challenge. The research requires caregivers, those diagnosed, and healthy individuals, but frequently, these opportunities are not relatively known. People may have various reasons for not wanting to participate in clinical research, which should be respected. However, one of my goals is to make sure one of those reasons is not a lack of information. This section will explore clinical trials from misconceptions, benefits, and risks to enrolling in clinical trials for people who feel prepared to fight the battle before and with us.

Phases of Drug Clinical Trials

Preclinical laboratory investigations provide scientific evidence that medicine is relatively safe and effective, but before the Food and Drug Administration (FDA) approves new medications for use. The drugs must complete a three-part clinical trial process (Phase I, II, and III). The new medicines must perform well enough in each phase before continuing to the next.

Phase I Trials

The first stage of human testing usually involves fewer than a hundred participants.

Healthy volunteers are usually present at this stage.

The tests are used to assess the risks and side effects of a drug.

Phase II Trials

A few hundred volunteers with the target condition participate in the second phase.

The studies are often too small to give convincing evidence about a treatment's benefit, but they provide additional information about safety and help determine the appropriate dosage of a medicine.

Phase III Trials

Hundreds to thousands of volunteers have enrolled in phase three studies, generally conducted at various study locations throughout the world.

They are the primary source of evidence for a drug's safety and efficacy that the FDA considers when deciding whether or not to approve it.

Phase IV Trials

The investigations are also known as post-marketing studies.

The FDA often requires phase four trials after the approval of a drug.

During this stage, scientists continue to track the health of people taking medicine to learn more about its long-term efficacy and safety.

Criteria to Participate

Not everyone can participate in a clinical trial: An individual must meet the study's eligibility requirements before enrolling in a clinical trial. All clinical trials have eligibility requirements for participants that researchers refer to as inclusion and exclusion criteria. Following are some examples of these criteria:

- Caregiver participation
- Disease stage
- Prescription drug use
- Age

- Other health conditions

Placebos

Scientists have learned that people sometimes feel better and even have improved results on medical tests when they *believe* a treatment is helping them, called the *placebo effect*. When a typical treatment plan for a condition is available, researchers often compare the experimental treatment to the standard treatment instead of using a placebo. Researchers often compare experimental treatment results to placebo results to determine new treatment efficacy.

There are two main strategies to reduce the likelihood that hope and belief will affect the outcome of clinical trials:

1. The trials are double-blinded, meaning neither the participants nor the researchers know who gets the experimental medication or the placebo.
2. Trials are placebo-controlled, meaning random participants get the experimental medication while others get an inactive pill, powder, or liquid called a placebo.

Clinical Trial Regulation

Solid regulations govern clinical trials for our protection, general order in the medical field, and strict compliance with ethical standards. The Food and Drug Administration is in charge of clinical trials, so doctors and science enthusiasts cannot just wake up one morning and start running clinical trials in their kitchens and garages.

Every clinical trial undertaken in the United States must first be approved by an Institutional Review Board (IRB). The IRB evaluates the trial's risk-benefit ratio and examines the trial protocols to ensure enough precautions are in place to ensure patient safety and that the experiment's stated objective is worthwhile.

IRBs are local, independent committees made up of community and patient advocates, researchers, physicians, and others who ensure that all clinical trials in their community adhere to acceptable standards and protect the study participants' rights and safety. The clinical trial design and execution teams comprise of doctors, scientists, researchers, nurses, pharmacists, medical writers, technicians, medical technologists, statisticians, secretarial, and support personnel. They each play an essential role in the progress of studies. Pharmaceutical firms, medical institutions, government organizations, charity foundations, and volunteering individuals or organizations fund clinical research to improve the future of medicine. Trials can occur in various settings such as universities, hospitals, doctors' offices, or community clinics.

Researchers often spend years studying and analyzing potential new medicines in laboratories, then they test the experimental treatments during animal studies before a clinical study that involves humans is allowed. The therapies that demonstrate the best results in these early laboratory studies are examined for human clinical trials.

With the FDA and IRBs doing their jobs to protect patients and other consumers, caregivers and family members can rest assured knowing that respectable clinical trials are there to help, not worsen. The choice remains up to the LOs and their families if they would like to participate in studies or not, and either decision is treated respectfully.

Informed Consent

Willingness is necessary to participate in clinical trials, but the FDA also requires that potential volunteers get comprehensive information regarding the study. Each potential participant meets a staff member for thorough explanations of the associated risks and potential benefits. After that, if they still want to proceed, participants must sign an informed consent form before participating in the trial and can decide to opt-out at any time.

Data Protection

Even though participants and research staff remain in the dark regarding who receives the test therapy and who receives the inactive placebo, most studies have a separate department that independently monitors trial information. The management committee members review data regularly and intervene if they discover any concerning patterns of adverse effects.

Researchers communicate important modifications to the study to keep all trial participants informed. While the early termination of a clinical trial may provoke powerful emotions in volunteers, it's crucial to remember that even if the outcome may not be positive, researchers have obtained vital data. Remember that clinical studies, including those that did not fulfill their expected results, gifted us with everything we now know about existing and promising treatments for Alzheimer's disease.

Patient Safety

The most crucial part of any Alzheimer's clinical research is patient safety. Each study's methods are assessed by an expert board not participating in the trial, which helps assure patient safety.

Benefits of Participation

Individuals who choose to participate in clinical trials are technically medical pioneers, and that label carries various benefits. They may, for example, obtain successful new therapies years before they are offered to the broader population. Clinical trial participants get the good stuff first. They assist others by participating in vital research that could lead to new treatments for certain diseases. Clinical trials give hope to folks diagnosed with Alzheimer's, their families, and generations. We all need something to hold on to, something to keep us going. While participating in the experiments, trial volunteers receive free expert medical treatment at major medical centers. However, remember that the benefits are limited to the research study, so LOs and their caregivers are still responsible for any medical care received outside the trial protocol.

Risks in Participation

Clinical trial participation is neither simple nor without risk. The consent form that participants (or their authorized caregivers) sign when they agree to participate in the clinical study spells out the hazards of participation.

Here are some disadvantages to consider:

The treatment may cause unpleasant or even possibly life-threatening side effects. One of the reasons why researchers perform clinical trials in the first place is to look for adverse effects. They must determine if the advantages of a particular treatment outweigh the hazards.

A study participant may go through the hustle of enrolling in a clinical study only to find out that the treatment is unsuccessful or that they were placed in the control group and never received the experimental medicine or therapy.

Clinical trial participation demands a significant time commitment.

Participants may be required to make repeated journeys to the study site, stay overnight in the hospital, and adhere to a strict diet or drug regimen.

Several healthcare providers may also see them during the study, especially if carried out at a big teaching hospital or research facility.

That can make families and friends feel like their LO is being treated like a test subject rather than a person.

Participants should also be aware that they must still seek treatment from their doctors if they have health problems unrelated to the trial's subject.

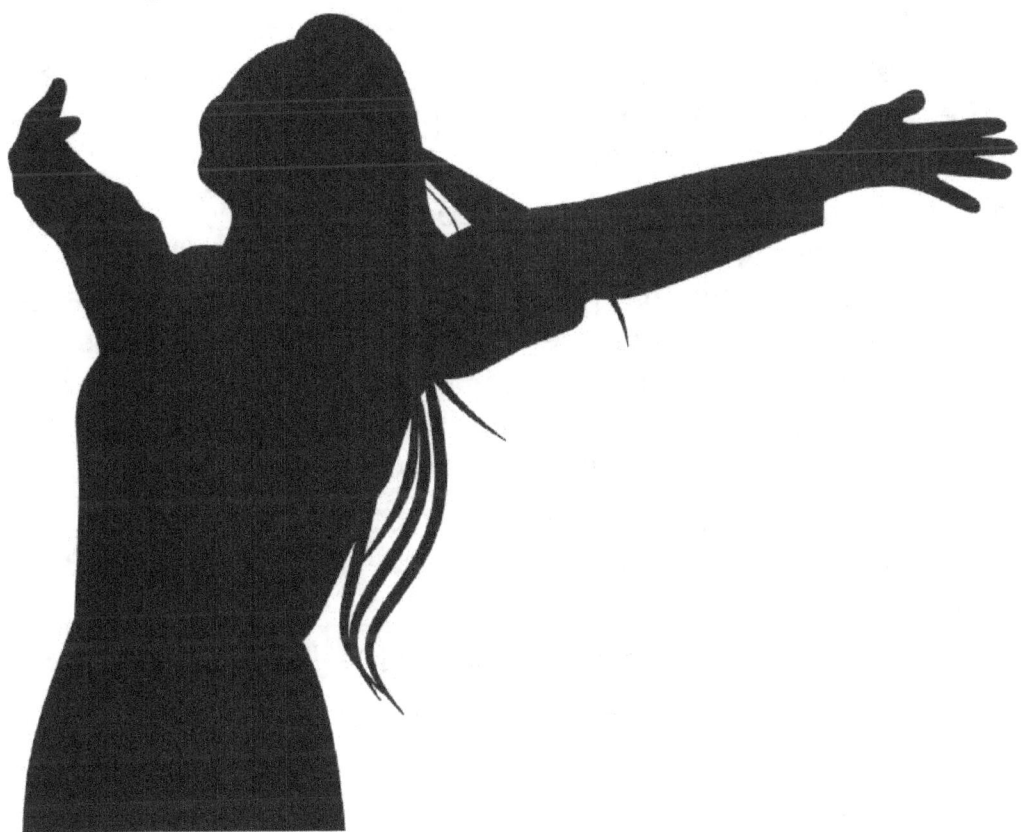

Optimism

Every new treatment that proceeds to clinical testing has to have convincing evidence that it will be as effective as or even more effective than currently available treatments. Whether or not the treatment performs as expected, every clinical trial adds to the body of knowledge. Even if the outcomes aren't encouraging, it's vital to remember that researchers have obtained valuable information.

Participating in clinical trials gives us hope for the now and the future. They make cutting-edge treatments and skilled medical care available to many people. They will eventually take us to the end of Alzheimer's disease.

Participants receive a high standard of care and oftentimes are given excellent opportunities to stand against the disease and fight alongside renowned scientists.

Participants receive excellent, ongoing care and have the opportunity to speak with clinical trial personnel. Regardless of trial results, research shows that people living with Alzheimer's disease who participate in clinical trials perform slightly better than those in a similar stage of their disease who do not participate in clinical trials. This advantage, scientists believe, is related to the generally excellent quality of care offered during clinical trials.

The federal government of the United States recommends that people considering participating in a clinical study ask the following questions:

- What is the objective of the study?
- Who will participate in the research?
- Why do scientists believe the new therapy being tested may be effective?
- Who will be responsible for my LO's care?
- Has it been tested before?
- How long will the trial last?
- What kinds of treatments and tests are involved?
- Will they need to stay in the hospital?

- How do the test medication's possible side effects and benefits compare with the current treatment?
- Will we receive the trial results?
- What type of long-term follow-up care is part of this study?
- Will we be reimbursed for other expenses?
- How might this trial affect their daily life?
- Who will pay for the treatment?
- How will we know that the treatment is working?

Individuals willing to participate in trials can find some of the answers to these concerns in the informed consent agreement, which all study participants must read and sign before entering a clinical trial. For further clarification, the researchers can provide any required information.

If there is anything I'd like you to take away from this section, an Alzheimer's diagnosis doesn't have to be your LO's fight alone; it's our fight, and together, we will get through this. I hope that one day we'll look back and say, "Remember when we had no cure for Alzheimer's?"

Chapter 8:

Creating Experiences

I just want to feel like I'm contributing. If you need anything, just call me; I can meal prep!

—Mom

Make the most out of the beautiful moments you spend with your LO. Create as many positive experiences as possible while piecing together some great memories.

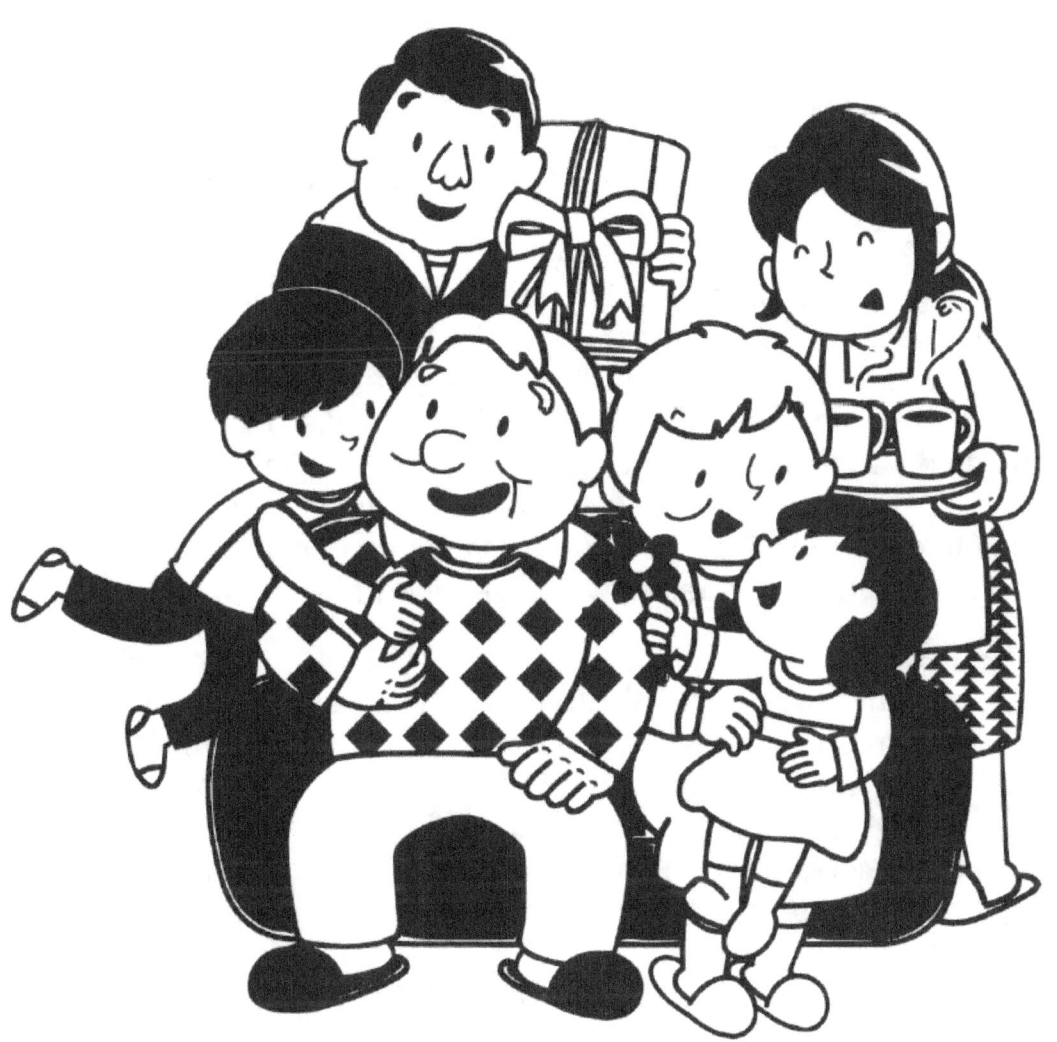

Try to make this time not all about running to doctor's appointments or feeling frustrated that your LO can no longer do the things that used to bring them joy in the past. This is an excellent time for you to relax and enjoy some momentary relief from the everyday stresses or even discover new joys.

Spending time with your LO promotes their happiness and cultivates yours in the long run. I found the following approaches helpful in my efforts to spend more quality time with your aging LOs.

Acceptance

Although our LOs may never be the same, they are still here. We have to approach and appreciate our interactions with understanding and acceptance of the reality of the disease.

Daily visits

Some caregivers admit having avoided constant interaction with their friend or family member with Alzheimer's disease because it hurts to see their LO fade. At the same time, they feel like there is nothing they can do about it. The fact is, there is. There is something you can do about it—be there with them. Your presence by their side makes a huge difference, so stop restraining yourself and let yourself feel. Try visiting your LO as much as possible and showing them nothing has changed how you see them.

Photo albums

Beautiful images communicate love, compassion, peace, and togetherness. They spread happiness and radiate warmth. Despite your LO's memory slowly fading away, a good photo from the past can nudge their memory to recollect the events leading to that pictured memory. Try going through family photo albums to pick the happiest pictures to remind your LO of their good old days. Fortunately, the 21st century offers many technological advancements that allow us to enjoy countless captured memories on digital platforms of our choice.

General Activities

Spending time with your LO is free and rewarding. Although many things come at a cost in this era, finding activities to involve your LO does not have to cost you a thing. There are several simple activities your LO might want to participate in, even without you having to leave the house. While these general activities may not improve your LO's memory, they are an easy way to create memories.

Cooking together

If your LO enjoys cooking, try joining them next time they are in the mood. You can also ask them to teach you some of their recipes. Your LO will feel that you really adore what they do, making them happy.

> **Story Time – Nope, I Got It!**
>
> My mom makes the best homemade biscuits in the world; songs have been written about her biscuits. Okay, perhaps that's not entirely true; many have commented favorably on her biscuits! She often offers to help with meal preparation. She refers to this as feeling "useful" or "pulling her weight" and "contributing to the household." I am certainly not perfect in this space. I used to decline help due to wanting to do everything for my mom or feeling like it would be quicker just to do it myself. I have learned this was working against me and becoming a missed opportunity to create more of those shared experiences.

Sharing media

Try sharing their favorite movies, music, and books. Make time for those childhood stories your LO may throw in after every movie scene that reminds them of their past. Try to show as much enthusiasm as you can because that will cheer them on, encouraging them to keep the conversation going.

Laundry

Your LO may have problems with colors or fabric textures but still offer to help with laundry. Sometimes, all you have to do is ask if they do not offer. Suggest the idea to them and see if they would be up for it. If they like the idea, sharing stories and creating memories while getting your household work done is a beautiful opportunity. You may realize that when you work together on activities such as laundry, even their usual confusion with colors or textures may seem as if it's gone—that is the magic of working together!

Try some of the following activities to improve the quality of time you spend with your LO.

Cleaning

If your LO once was a perfectionist, the type that offers to clean your bathroom because you cannot do it right, chances are they want to show you how they like the kitchen cleaned, so invite them to help! If the diagnosed is your parent, they have a way they like to do things. However, they may not always tell you, so when you suggest activities such as cleaning together, you get a chance to create memories and allow them to teach you. Science says that's how best we learn, so try not to worry about how often your LO will show you how to clean the stove after use.

Gardening

Did your LO have a garden before their diagnosis? There is no reason to stop now! Their flowers and herbs do not have to wilt when you can take care of them together. While your LO would also appreciate the change of scenery, the scents and colors of their favorite flowers can unlock beautiful memories from their past. Ask them to help you water their garden plants, arrange flowers, or grow fruits. There are a lot of activities you can do in the garden to help your LO open up more while having memorable moments.

Physical Activities

Regular physical exercise is among the most critical activities your LO can do to improve fitness. Frequent physical activity helps slow down and even prevent several health problems accompanying the aging process. Exercise also aids muscle growth, enabling your LO to continue carrying out tasks independently for a longer time than they would without physical activity.

You can try spending some of your free time exploring your LO's physical routine. Having a partner makes exercise more enjoyable, but more than that, you can make it memorable with your LO!

Your LO might love some of the following activities:

Dancing

Does your LO like stretching their legs and moving around? If so, they might enjoy dancing too. Dancing is a great way to blow steam while exercising. Different people prefer different dances depending on their body type, mood on the day in question, and many other reasons. The other thing I love about dancing is that one can dance when in high spirits, and they can also dance the stress out of a bad day. Perfect, right?

Walking

If dancing seems to use up more energy than is on the table, you can suggest short walks around your home, neighborhood, or the local farmers' market. The weather may determine how much walking you will do because you are likely to tire easily if it is hot. If the atmosphere is cool and inviting, embark upon new adventures together and explore all that your neighborhood has to offer.

Yoga

A calm workout for slow weekends, yoga can help you, and your LO lets go of your previous week's stress and refocus on your relationship and other important matters in preparation for a brand-new week. It is suitable for flexibility and balance and can help your LO relieve back pain. Try suggesting yoga to your LO and wait to see if they would be up for the idea. You can even take classes together if your LO feels like interacting with other people.

Swimming

Perfect for hot days, swimming is another activity you can take on with your LO. It is an excellent low-impact activity that can help build muscle strength, allowing you to relax. Ask your LO if they would be interested in swimming.

Gym

You can also try light exercises at the gym. Ask your LO if they would like to exercise with you. If you have a gym at home, you can even accompany the exercise with your LO's favorite music, as long as the tempo is suitable for your workouts. If you have to go out to the gym, make sure your instructor knows and understands your LO's situation, sharing just enough details as appropriate. The instructor might even suggest other exercises you can try with your LO. If your LO is not worried about meeting new people, this can also be an opportunity to meet other people in similar situations.

Night-time Activities

If you carefully pick suitable nighttime activities with your LO, you reduce the chances of them interrupting your sleep later at night after they fail to rest, get scared, or think it's already morning.

Although your relationship with your LO determines the appropriateness of your chosen activities, whichever plan you draw should have a soothing effect.

Strenuous activities may be unsuitable for nights as it is time for your LO to relax before drifting to their dreamland. Some of the following activities may help your LO sleep better at night.

Massage

Have you noticed how a calm back rub can ease a crying baby to sleep? Apply a similar skill here and watch it work like sleep magic. I, of course, understand your exact relationship with the patient determines your choice of techniques for nighttime massages, so find whatever works for your situation.

While a simple hand or foot massage can do, you can make it more sensual if the LO is your spouse. That gives you a chance to soothe your LO to sleep while reconnecting with them. Even if the LO is your husband, men love massages too, so do not be afraid to challenge yourself.

Aromatherapy

If you try massages and your LO enjoys them, you can blend in some scents to awaken their sense of smell. You can make use of essential oils or scented candles during your massages. Be cautious about allergies and avoid scents your LO does not seem to enjoy. Aromatherapy is relaxing and helps alleviate stress as well as anxiety. It can also unlock some of your LO's memories, which are all significant wins.

Teas

Try making bedtime tea together. Teas such as lavender or chamomile help improve sleep quality. If your LO enjoys working in the kitchen, they might be thrilled to share more soothing teas and how to make them. Some types of teas have traditions surrounding their origin, and if your LO used to have an interest in such subjects, they might welcome a chance to become a professor in one night!

Letters

Depending on how fast the disease worsens, you can find writing letters very useful to calm your LO down before they sleep. Some patients who experience confusion may have trouble sleeping because they miss someone, a long-lost friend, a spouse, or a child. When your LO misses people who are no longer within reach, you can employ a technique called *therapeutic lying* to relax their mind. Therapeutic lying is a communication technique that gives you a temporary ticket into your LO's reality, to actively participate in a conversation during their episodes of confusion without confusing them further. An example is if your divorced parents said they missed their spouse. If that thought seems to keep interfering with their inner peace, you can tap into their world and suggest writing their LO a letter regardless of intentions to actually deliver it.

Breathing

Another effective technique to help your LO sleep better at night while you spend memorable time together is to try breathing exercises. Although breathing may not present many chances for connection, it increases your chances of getting good, uninterrupted sleep at bedtime.

Family Activities

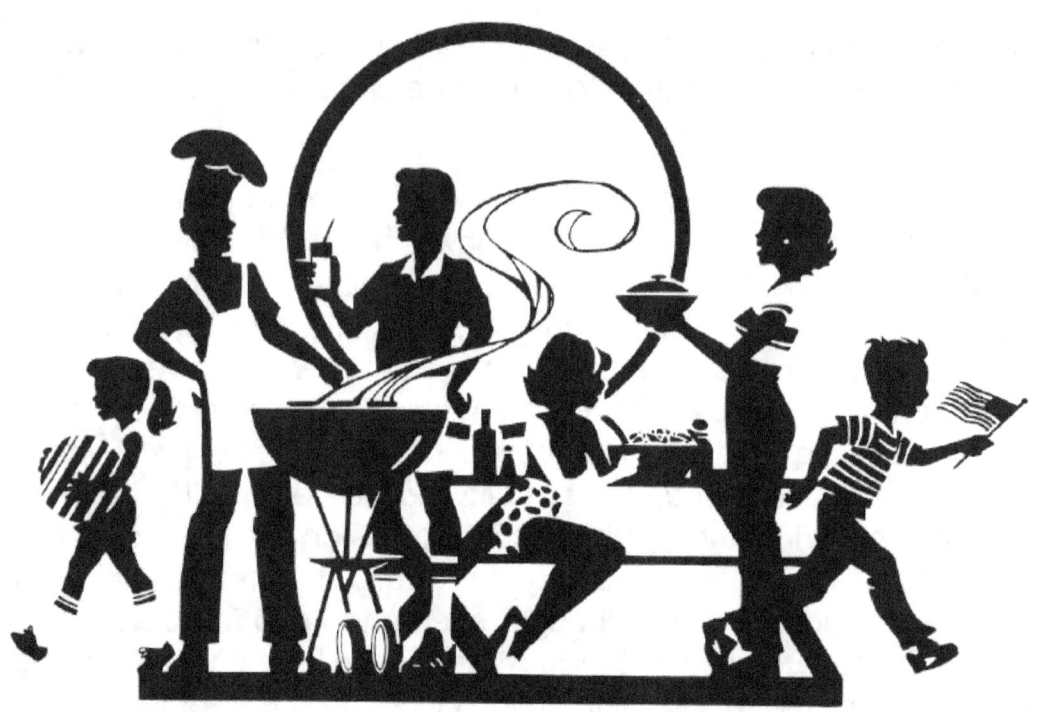

Just as you don't have to do this without a care team, you don't have to do it without family either! Try discussing how important it is to frequently interact with your LO with your family. Nothing warms a parent's heart more than seeing their children happy together. If the diagnosed is your parent or grandparent, invite your siblings over when they are free and organize family dates once in a while. If the patient is your spouse, friend, or in some cases, child, invite their close friends and family over for a home-cooked meal or something even more special. Make it count.

You might want to try activities that promote interaction, such as:

Family barbecue

It is a beautiful sight to have family members together for feasting activities such as barbecuing or good old family dinners. If sharing food and fuel can bring nations together, sharing food and stories surely can bring families together! Although your LO would appreciate you inviting family over for special family time, remember to check in with them first. It may not end well if you invite people that your LO would rather avoid or if you surprise them on a bad day.

Scrapbooking

In the depths of confusion, when all else ceases to make sense, we can still find the strength to focus on a scrapbook. Scrapbooking gives your LO a chance to showcase their imagination in a peaceful environment. Because it is a less challenging task, they get a sense of satisfaction knowing they fulfilled a task without much difficulty. Doing this with family makes it even more rewarding because you can all enjoy the stories behind each picture or drawing. Even if your family is far away and you cannot make it in person, technology has your back. You can use video conferencing platforms such as Zoom and get everyone there with the click of a link. Problem solved.

Date night

If the LO is your spouse, keep the spirit high by surprising your partner with a well-arranged date night. It does not have to cost a small fortune. Depending on the mood you want to set and whether your LO is an indoor person or the adventurous, outgoing type, you can even set it up in your backyard.

Taking pictures

You can make your special family gatherings more memorable by capturing the moments in pictures. Photos live to tell stories when we forget or are no longer there to share bits and pieces behind each of them. They are a fabulous way to remember the beautiful moments you can cherish with your LO forever. You can even suggest having professional photoshoots once in a while, but don't underestimate the power of a good, optimally timed selfie!

Community work

Chances are your LO wants to remain helpful. If they like helping others, suggest a volunteer activity you can do together, such as soup kitchens or animal shelters. You'll get the dual benefit of creating memories together AND helping your community. It can offer a temporary reprieve from your collective worries.

Family adventures

Does your LO like traveling? If they are the kind that gets bored by being in one place for long, then they might like the idea of going on an adventure as a family. Suggest going to places they enjoy and give them time to think about it. Do not be discouraged if your LO is not up for the idea; remember that some individuals may want to avoid crowds and new places. Even if your LO has already been to a particular place, sometimes it may feel new and confusing to them.

Food for the Mind

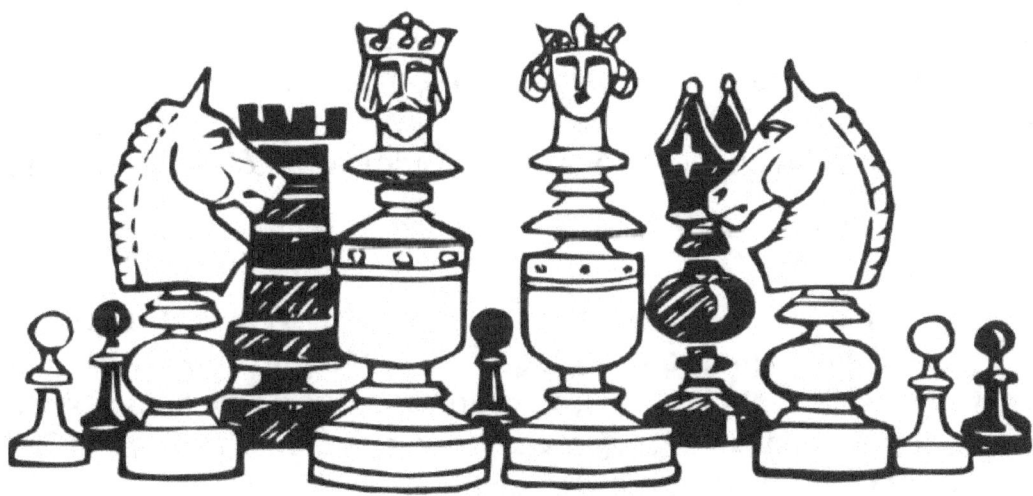

The human brain benefits from what we feed our bodies and the mental activities we engage in. With our LOs, the mind is already going through too much for us to starve it, so we need to help our LOs by encouraging activities that improve memory and other cognitive skills. Activities that challenge your LO while giving you quality time include:

Solving puzzles

Jigsaw puzzles are an excellent way to spend time with your LO while exercising their brain. They are ideal because they have different difficulty levels, so you can choose based on your LO's mood or the concentration level they have that day. These games can also include vocabulary games, word puzzles, or sudoku.

Art and crafts

If your LO is artistic and constantly working on creative projects, you can share in their joy by offering to help. From sculpting to knitting and recycling old bottles into fountains, investing time in art and crafts rewards the mind, body, and soul. Your LO might even have a skill or two to show you, so this can be a learning opportunity for you, too!

Suppose your LO is not interested in activities that take time to complete. In that case, you can suggest more specific activities to decorate the home, such as framed pictures, a drawing to hang on the wall, or making changes to any other item your LO would want to beautify.

Playing card games

Your LO might enjoy playing card games if they like devising strategies. Card games are an ideal opportunity to unwind after a long week while your LO sharpens their mind. They help relieve stress, improve patience, and revamp their strategic thinking skills. Ask your LO if they would be interested in playing card games with you.

Singing

Behind every one of your LO's favorite songs is a story waiting for you to unlock it. Like dancing, songs can work when your LO is in a poor mood. Ask them to sing you their favorite songs and join in. Going through the lyrics in their mind helps improve their thinking skills, so you can even ask them to write the lyrics for you and assess their work. You may be surprised; your LO may joyously remember every last word from a favorite song from decades ago while, in the same instant, having difficulties remembering a conversation from five minutes prior.

Online games

Is your LO tech-savvy and would rather play digital games? Find self-care memory games you can play with your LO and invite them to challenge you. Mark the games they enjoy the most and take note of the ones they seem to dislike so you know what to suggest in the future.

Playing chess

If you can get your LO to play chess with you, it improves their concentration and fuels critical thinking. If they win without feeling like you deliberately skewed the odds in their favor, knowing they can still beat a mentally healthy person boosts their self-confidence and encourages them to play again next time. Some individuals may dislike the idea of chess because it can be difficult to master if one is only a learner.

Interacting With Caution

As you try to create memories with your LO, avoid letting the enthusiasm sweep you off your current reality. Remember that your LO still has difficulties, and some activities may be uncomfortable for them. What follows are some points to remember.

Remember that although you are the one who will remember your shared experiences in the long term, this is still about your LO. Consider letting them lead and pay attention to their concerns. Try to be as agreeable as possible if your LO suggests a different activity because they don't feel like participating in the other one.

Opt for activities that give them purpose or deliver a direct benefit. Consider explaining why you would want to participate in their activities whenever you offer help with activities. They may consider personal, such as painting their favorite scenery or writing letters to their LO. They will perform the activity better when they know what it offers, and thorough explanations also help reduce their chances of turning you down. Our LOs tend to grow suspicious, so they may wonder about your secret agenda if you just pop up behind them and offer to help them read their old letters or any personal documents.

Your LO will repeatedly tell you the same stories, and there is nothing much to do about it. They may also suggest the same activities or games because they enjoy them. Try to avoid saying things like:

- "You already told me that story."
- "How many times do we have to watch the same thing?"

Following your LO's lead does not mean you should listen to music from the beginning of time and pretend to enjoy it while you silently die inside. If you would instead do something else with your LO, or if you feel you have had enough of one activity, story, or game, consider saying something like the following:

- "Would you like to play something else today?"
- "I found something interesting you will enjoy!"
- "Would you like to continue tomorrow?"

The key is understanding. Try listening to yourself from their standpoint. If you did not sound polite enough, learn and try again next time. If you were unconvincing, practice speaking with confidence and try again. If you feel you did everything right, but it's just them, take a breath, smile, and make it worth your while. It is part of the journey.

Conclusion

You have reached the beginning of your new normal. Getting this far is unparalleled proof of your determination to do the most for your LO. Note that this book's healthcare and legal information is advice for a friend from a friend. I do not intend to mislead; the information in this book should not be treated as professional medical or legal advice. For guidance, find reputable institutions and professionals who can provide the most accurate and up-to-date information.

In This Book we discussed Alzheimer's disease and other forms of dementia to clearly understand what normal aging is and what it is not. In subsequent chapters, we tackled problems you may face as a caregiver, the sacrifices that await you, and explored what you can do to overcome caregiving difficulties. Because communication is a significant challenge for many patients and caregivers, we also covered various strategies to help you get the most out of your appointments with healthcare professionals. In later chapters, we discussed how you can accept your new reality and draw strength to move forward. It is essential that you appreciate the importance of your role, even when no one says anything about it.

I also shared quotes from my mom and personal stories to help you relate and understand that we have the same fight and will get through this together. Although you have reached the end of this book, it comforts me to know you can always refer back to specific chapters that you need to understand more.

I hope you find peace knowing there is hope for our LOs and ourselves. Change may take time, but we should remain confident we are doing the best for all those involved. If you found this book useful, you can share it with a friend and help spread the information. If you enjoyed this read, feel free to let me know by leaving an honest review on Amazon.

References

Alzheimer's Association. (2019). *Vascular Dementia*. Alzheimer's Disease and Dementia. https://www.alz.org/alzheimers-dementia/what-is-dementia/types-of-dementia/vascular-dementia

Alzheimer's Association. (2021a). *How clinical trials work*. Alzheimer's Disease and Dementia. https://www.alz.org/alzheimers-dementia/research_progress/clinical-trials/how-trials-work

Alzheimer's Association. (2021b). *Why participate in a clinical trial*? Alzheimer's Disease and Dementia. https://www.alz.org/alzheimers-dementia/research_progress/clinical-trials/why-participate

Bernstein, S. (2007). *What Is Lewy Body Dementia*? WebMD. https://www.webmd.com/alzheimers/guide/dementia-lewy-bodies

Cummings, J., Aisen, P., Apostolova, L. G., Atri, A., Salloway, S., & Weiner, M. (2021). Aducanumab: Appropriate use recommendations. *The Journal of Prevention of Alzheimer's Disease, 1–13*. https://doi.org/10.14283/jpad.2021.41

Davis, S. (2016, September 12). *What's Normal Aging*? WebMD; WebMD. https://www.webmd.com/healthy-aging/guide/normal-aging

DeNoon, D. J. (2009, October 1). *7 Stages of Alzheimer's Disease*. WebMD; WebMD. https://www.webmd.com/alzheimers/guide/alzheimers-disease-stages

Drugs.com (2019). *Aging overview.* Drugs. https://www.drugs.com/health-guide/aging.html

Fidelity Life. (n.d.). *What is a simplified issue life insurance policy?* Fidelity Life. Retrieved May 2022, from https://fidelitylife.com/learn-and-plan/learning-center/types-of-life-insurance/simplified-issue-life/#:~:text=What%20is%20simplified%20issue%20insurance

Hicks, P. (n.d.). *Estate planning 101: What is estate planning?* Trust & Will. https://trustandwill.com/learn/what-is-estate-planning

Laird, L. (n.d.). *Will vs. trust: What's the difference?* Www.legalzoom.com. Retrieved May 2022, from https://www.legalzoom.com/articles/will-vs-trust-whats-the-difference

Learn about clinical studies. (n.d.). Clinicaltrials.gov. https://www.clinicaltrials.gov/ct2/about-studies/learn

Lethin, C., Leino-Kilpi, H., Bleijlevens, M. H., Stephan, A., Martin, M. S., Nilsson, K., Nilsson, C., Zabalegui, A., & Karlsson, S. (2018). Predicting caregiver burden in informal caregivers caring for persons with dementia living at home – A follow-up cohort study. *Dementia,* 19(3), 640–660. https://doi.org/10.1177/1471301218782502

Martindale-Adams, J., Nichols, L. O., Zuber, J., Burns, R., & Graney, M. J. (2015). Dementia Caregivers' Use of Services for Themselves. *The Gerontologist,* 56(6), 1053–1061. https://doi.org/10.1093/geront/gnv121

Mayo Clinic. (n.d.). *What to know about the stages of Alzheimer's.* Mayo Clinic. https://www.mayoclinic.org/diseases-conditions/alzheimers-disease/in-depth/alzheimers-stages/art-20048448#:~:text=There%20are%20five%20stages%20associated

Mayo Clinic. (2018). *Vascular dementia - Symptoms and causes*. Mayo Clinic. https://www.mayoclinic.org/diseases-conditions/vascular-dementia/symptoms-causes/syc-20378793

National Institute on Aging. (n.d.). *What is Lewy body dementia? Causes, symptoms, and treatments*. National Institute on Aging. https://www.nia.nih.gov/health/what-lewy-body-dementia-causes-symptoms-and-treatments#:~:text=Lewy%20body%20dementia%20(LBD)%20is

National Institute on Aging. (2018). *How is Alzheimer's disease treated?* National Institute on Aging. https://www.nia.nih.gov/health/how-alzheimers-disease-treated

National Institute on Aging. (2021, July 2). *What Is Dementia? Symptoms, Types, and Diagnosis*. National Institute on Aging. https://www.nia.nih.gov/health/what-is-dementia

Smith, P. B., Kenan, M., & Kunik, M. E. (2004). *Alzheimer's for dummies*. Wiley Publishing.

Steenfeldt, V. Ø., Aagerup, L. C., Jacobsen, A. H., & Skjødt, U. (2021). Becoming a Family Caregiver to a Person with Dementia: A Literature Review on the Needs of Family Caregivers. *SAGE Open Nursing, 7*, 237796082110290. https://doi.org/10.1177/23779608211029073

WebMD. (2011, October 10). *Treatments for Alzheimer's disease*. WebMD. https://www.webmd.com/alzheimers/guide/alzheimers-disease-treatment-overview

Image Sources

AnnaliseArt. (2019, June 1). *Family*. Pixabay. https://cdn.pixabay.com/photo/2019/06/02/12/42/family-4246393_960_720.png

ArtsyBeeKids. (2020, October 18). *Gavel mallet icon*. Pixabay. https://cdn.pixabay.com/photo/2020/10/16/19/22/gavel-5660494_960_720.png

Clker. (2012a, April 2). *Ambulance*. Pixabay. https://cdn.pixabay.com/photo/2012/04/02/12/50/ambulance-24405_960_720.png

Clker. (2012b, April 11). *Medication taking hand*. Pixabay. https://cdn.pixabay.com/photo/2012/04/13/00/06/medication-31119_960_720.png

Clker. (2012c, April 17). *BBQ party outdoors*. Pixabay. https://cdn.pixabay.com/photo/2012/04/18/01/22/bbq-36427_960_720.png

Dapple Designers. (2019, September 27). *Medical hospital icons*. Pixabay. https://cdn.pixabay.com/photo/2019/09/28/10/38/medical-4510408_960_720.png

Elf-Moondance. (2021, September 27). *Memory loss*. Pixabay. https://cdn.pixabay.com/photo/2021/09/25/03/24/alzheimers-disease-6653912_960_720.jpg

GDJ. (2022, February 4). *Mental health*. Pixabay. https://cdn.pixabay.com/photo/2022/02/04/02/32/mental-health-6991769_960_720.png

Geralt. (2015, July 1). *Caregiver*. Pixabay. https://cdn.pixabay.com/photo/2015/06/30/08/29/dependent-826332_960_720.jpg

Geralt. (2017a, March 27). *Teamwork*. Pixabay. https://cdn.pixabay.com/photo/2017/03/30/11/12/teamwork-2188038_960_720.jpg

Geralt. (2017b, June 28). *Together*. Pixabay. https://cdn.pixabay.com/photo/2017/06/28/08/28/together-2450090_960_720.jpg

Geralt. (2018, March 26). *Alzheimer's*. Pixabay. https://cdn.pixabay.com/photo/2018/03/28/07/51/dementia-3268560_960_720.jpg

Geralt. (2019, March 13). *Dance yoga meditation*. Pixabay. https://cdn.pixabay.com/photo/2019/03/13/12/38/dance-4052847_960_720.jpg

Hassan, M. (2017, August 24). *Nurse old woman*. Pixabay. https://cdn.pixabay.com/photo/2017/08/26/17/54/nurse-2683782_960_720.png

Hassan, M. (2018, July 28). *Feel free*. Pixabay. https://cdn.pixabay.com/photo/2018/07/27/18/13/feel-free-3566550_960_720.png

Hassan, M. (2022, May 16). *Nursing*. Pixabay. https://cdn.pixabay.com/photo/2022/05/15/10/43/nursing-7197237_960_720.png

OpenClipart. (2016a, March 19). *Elderly families*. Pixabay. https://cdn.pixabay.com/photo/2016/03/31/22/02/children-1296800_960_720.png

OpenClipart. (2016b, March 30). *Black and white chess game*. Pixabay. https://cdn.pixabay.com/photo/2016/04/01/00/09/black-and-white-1298024_960_720.png

Rexazin, M. (2020, August 4). *Medical health*. Pixabay. https://cdn.pixabay.com/photo/2020/08/03/09/39/medical-5459633_960_720.png

Tumisu. (2018, April 20). *Mental health*. Pixabay. https://cdn.pixabay.com/photo/2018/04/20/20/57/mental-health-3337018_960_720.jpg

www.ingramcontent.com/pod-product-compliance
Lightning Source LLC
Chambersburg PA
CBHW062106220526
45471CB00010B/3623